"Parenting will never be easy. ̣... ̣...... ̣... ̣ ...... ̣ing, enjoyable, and effective with the right mind-set and communication strategies. Raising Healthy Parents is a sane, funny, and eminently practical guide to the journey of a lifetime. If your parenting could use an infusion of joy, clarity, and compassion, Sid is your guide, and Raising Healthy Parents is your user's manual."

HOWARD JACOBSON, PHD, host of *The Plant Yourself Podcast*, contributing author to *Proteinaholic* and *Whole*

"Small Steps for the win! For achieving a healthier, happier family, you've found the best approach for creating lasting change and the best person you could have chosen to be your guide on this journey."

MATT FRAZIER, author of *No Meat Athlete* and *The No Meat Athlete Cookbook*

"A fun, easy-to-read, practical parenting book that cuts the crap and gimmicks to focus on the real goal: happiness. Sid Garza-Hillman's approach centers around becoming a happy and well-balanced parent, and, in turn, raising healthy, thriving, and yes, happy children. A must-read for new parents like myself."

DOUG HAY, founder of *Rock Creek Runner* and cohost of *No Meat Athlete Radio*

"As parents, we are inundated with information about how to raise our children but receive little, if any, guidance on how to raise ourselves. Healthy, active, well-adjusted parents are more resilient and better suited to the task of child-rearing and LIFE. Sid Garza-Hillman walks us through the process of achieving this end in a practical, realistic, no BS way."

AARON STUBER & **JACKSON LONG** of *Thought For Food Lifestyle*

"'Parenting is an imperfect art.' It's not about following the latest model for modifying children's behaviors; it's about the parents. In his charismatic tone, Sid sets an example for parents to first understand more about themselves in order to build a healthy family. Whether your children are just a glimmer in your eye or getting ready to flee the nest, this is a must-read that will create a positive transformation for you, your home, and your family."

ADAM & **SHOSHANA CHAIM,** cohosts of *The Plant Trainers Podcast*

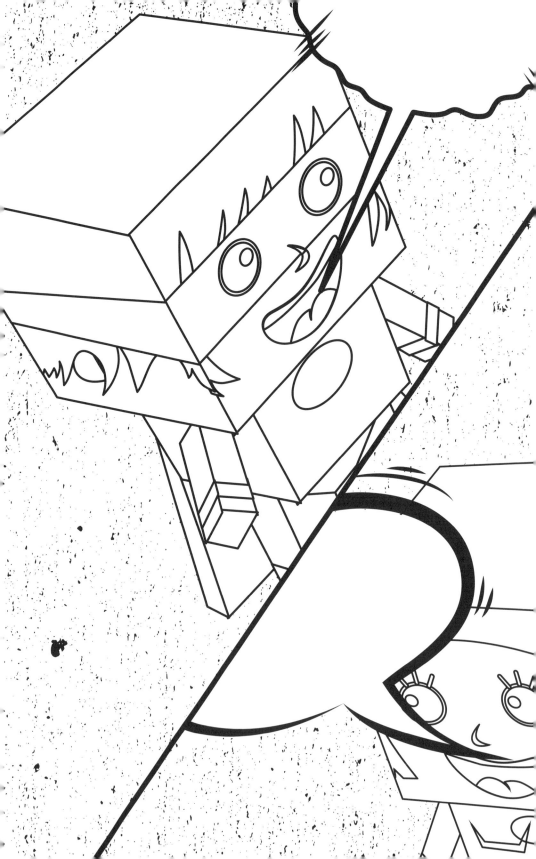

RAISING

HEALTHY

PARENTS

SID GARZA-HILLMAN

Foreword by Matt Frazier, the No Meat Athlete

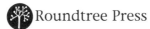 Roundtree Press

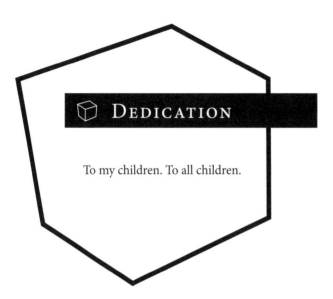

DEDICATION

To my children. To all children.

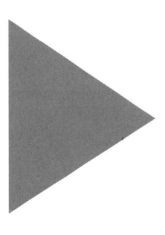

LET'S

TAKE A MOMENT

Pause

CONTENTS

FOREWORD
by Matt Frazier

PREFACE

INTRODUCTION

THE REST OF THE BOOK.

FOREWORD

It's easier than ever to be a parent . . . just like it's easier than ever to nourish ourselves with food.

Start with the food. We live in an era of unprecedented nutritional convenience, where thousands of calories sit waiting to be consumed in airtight packages, right in our pantries. Should we find those options unsatisfactory, our next meal is only a short drive away at a local fast-food spot (no need to even get out of the car). And those times we're feeling really lazy, it only takes a few taps on the smartphone to ask for hot food to be delivered right to our door.

A far cry from having to grow, gather, or hunt our food. Oh, and then having to eat it in the short window before it spoils. And, sometimes, not to be able to eat at all for a few hours. Or even a few days.

And yet, for all the ease of nourishing ourselves in today's world, we're fatter and sicker than we've ever been—I mean, like, global epidemic level.

Similarly, technology makes it easier than ever to be a parent. One need only search YouTube for "kids show 3 hours" to find exactly that (yes, they put the length right in the title for you). The cheapest babysitter on the planet, and she's available on short notice . . . even on weekends.

Long car ride? Bring the tablets. (If the screens aren't already installed in the seats, of course.)

Thanks to the miracle of modern technology—and that food bit we already talked about—it's conceivable that one could raise kids that survive without ever having to see or hear them, once they're old enough to swipe and pinch. (Which, if you've ever had the astonishing experience of watching a toddler navigate an iPhone, you know isn't very old.)

Yep . . . easier than ever.

While we're starting to get a clear picture of what the convenience-food lifestyle does to our health, the impact of digital babysitting remains to be seen. But do we really have to wonder how it'll turn out?

In his first book, *Approaching the Natural*—one of my favorites, that I've given to (literally) hundreds of people—Sid Garza-Hillman argues that we need only look to nature to discover the optimal ways to eat, move, and live for long-term health and short-term happiness.

We all agree that in the modern world it's not always practical to go barefoot and forage for our food. But if we can only approach this ideal, say, by buying fresh produce and moving our bodies more often, then we're making a dramatically better choice than the current default, without going full-caveman.

And it's exactly the same when it comes to parenting. Just like our bodies have evolved to thrive on real, actual food—the only way we used to be able to eat, period—our kids' minds (and bodies, too) are optimized for the way kids used to be raised. I don't mean the "good ol' days," with a white picket fence, dinner at 5:00 PM sharp, and stickball in the vacant lot down the street until then. I mean much, much further back than that: the caveman days. But remember, we only need to approach the ideal to find the sweet spot between modern and optimal that best allows us (and our children) to thrive in today's world.

I have two children, a boy and girl, aged seven and four as I write this. And because my wife and I have raised them while coming to understand the "approaching the natural" way of thinking about food, it has been fairly easy to make the leap and allow this philosophy to extend into our parenting.

My children both eat a healthy diet, even though they understand that they have a choice in the matter. How do we get them to make good choices? Actually, it's been surprisingly stress-free. My wife and I talk to them often about why we choose to eat this way; they help in the garden and even, now and then, in making foods like fresh pasta from scratch. They understand where food comes from, and their taste buds haven't been blasted with artificial flavors or unnaturally sweet, salty, or fatty foods.

 If the opportunity to eat a way-less-than-healthy cupcake at a school birthday party presents itself and no healthier option is available, they understand they can do what they want. (And what they want, almost always, is the choice to eat the way they do when they're with us.)

This is our way of approaching what we think is pretty darn natural, without making them go dig up a sweet potato from the ground every day for lunch. And in staying flexible, we hopefully avoid most situations where they need to feel stress or, even worse, guilt.

To take another example, until just a few weeks ago my kids slept in the same room. It wasn't that we didn't have the space for separate rooms; instead, we wanted them to be able to hear and take comfort in the sound of another human being breathing when they woke up at night in the dark. The way it used to be, by default.

Some days—okay, most days, since pretty much every time one wakes up, the other does too—that hasn't felt easy. But when we see them play together, respect each other, and love each other, the choice to embrace the inconvenience feels worth it.

My kids play sports. They do art. They even meditate. And yes, sometimes they play video games. We have boundaries, and they respect them. So how do you raise kids who are athletic, artistic, respectful, patient, determined, mindful—and still normal?

Easy. By being those things yourself and making those traits the very air that your kids breathe. But this isn't the same "easy" as convenience food and screentime. And that's where Sid can help. Maybe you've heard that clichéd, favorite adage of parenting books about "putting your own oxygen mask on first."

It means you can only effectively parent if you've already taken care of your own needs. It contains a kernel of truth, of course, but if your version of an oxygen mask mostly looks like three beers a night and a whole lot of Netflix, then putting it on first won't do you or your kids much good in the long run.

This is what *Raising Healthy Parents* is all about. Instead of the beers and movie-streaming sites, your oxygen mask is healthy food, lots of movement, meaningful hobbies, time with friends, and the like. The stuff that feels great once you start doing it, but isn't the easiest choice when you're stressed or used to a different set of habits.

But changing habits around health is where Sid shines. While the *Biggest Loser* culture loves to highlight the motivational drill sergeant pushing her subject's willpower to the breaking point, Sid tells his clients to "start with a glass of water" or "add a stalk of celery to your dinner" as a first step. Only when that tiny bit of progress becomes your new normal, do you take the next small step.

His approach is for his clients to first build trust in their own abilities to follow through, nurturing and growing their willpower over time, rather than existing under the perfectionist illusion of overnight transformation—only to have it come crashing down in spectacular fashion when it all becomes too much.

In the meal plan program we run together, Health Made Simple, Sid and I regularly counsel new members who beat themselves up for "falling off the wagon" when they try to follow a plan, against our advice, to perfection the first week. This, of course, is the downside of perfectionism—the shame that comes from failure, and the mental and emotional effort to pick up the pieces and start again. Until eventually, it becomes easier to stop trying altogether.

But what if, as Sid and I now teach, there were no wagon? What if there were no falling off, and, instead, only the recognition that a certain meal, workout, or interaction with your kids didn't go as well as it might have? What if there were an understanding that what matters isn't any single episode, but instead what you do *most of the time* (your "MOTT," as Sid calls it)?

Then there would be no shame around supposed failure. In fact, short of completely giving up on your desired outcome, there would be no failure at all—and that all-too-familiar experience of throwing in the towel in frustration is exactly what Sid's approach is so great at preventing.

This is the beauty of Sid's philosophy, and why I'm so excited that you've placed your trust in him by picking up this book. The "small steps" approach—to eating, moving, parenting, and anything else—takes time and patience, both of which are in exceedingly short supply these days. But its power for creating change is unmatched, and when its legions of devotees grows, the world becomes better for it. You've found the best approach for creating lasting change, and the best person you could have chosen to be your guide on this journey.

—MATT FRAZIER

FACE PRE
PREFACE
FACE PRE

began writing this book on Thanksgiving weekend. Whatever this holiday's history, Thanksgiving has come to mean time with family and an expression of gratitude. Seems the perfect time to begin a book about healthy and happy families. I believe that most modern humans, if stripped of all technology, music, movies, books, and transportation, would be profoundly thankful just to have their families and friends with them. We find true, long-term happiness through our relationships. We are wired this way, and our tribes can support and fulfill us. We understand this because it is how we have evolved.

With all the "social" technology at our fingertips, including Skype and FaceTime, there still is no substitute for actually being *with* our families—parents, children, siblings, grandparents, and, of course, our chosen families: our friends. My hope is to empower parents to grab more joy from the little time we have with our children before they head out into the world to raise their own families.

It is in this spirit that I began writing this book. The spirit of family. The spirit of connection. What we hold most dear. With all the different parenting/family approaches, it's easy to lose sight of what we are really trying to do—eke out a happy life, a life that is full of joy, of meaning, of fulfillment. With that goal as our backdrop, we are better able to make changes and adjustments when and if necessary. We don't dig our heels in and continue with behaviors that no longer serve us or our families, because it becomes less about what is happening in the moment and more about the bigger picture. By placing our happiness above all else, we'll adjust, change, adapt to do whatever it takes to raise the happiest, healthiest families we can.

It is raining outside as I write this. My seven-year-old twins have just exclaimed that they have nothing to do. All this while standing in a room filled with books, games, Legos, art supplies, blocks, cars, and trains. Two pieces of aluminum foil later, boats are built, raincoats are on, and adventure lives another day. In a world where we have access to an unprecedented amount of entertainment, an unlikely solution to boredom sometimes means getting back to basics.

Twenty minutes later, one of the twins comes in to report a series of scenarios she has just created—she built another boat, made yet another from tree bark, and found several places to float them. Simultaneously, the other twin comes in to make sure I was super clear about the utter ridiculousness of even suggesting that creating and floating foil boats is anything but a useless endeavor. On any other day, I might easily get the opposite reactions from each. Such is the unpredictable nature of families . . .

Three hours later, we can't get the kids to sleep. We want a frickin' moment to ourselves before we go to bed. We're trying to finish some work we couldn't get to during the day because of the every-third-minute interruption that happens as if timed on a stopwatch. As we yet again tell them to go to sleep, we watch ourselves (almost like we're watching a movie) turn into creatures of the underworld. Our voices literally morph into a combination of Gollum's and Sam Kinison's. We "lose ourselves" and later, in a daze of fatigue, feel bad about what went down.

Parenting is an imperfect art. There is neither one fixed approach nor one-size-fits-all actions. No two families are alike, in the same way that no two people are alike. However, I wanted to write a book to help people understand that familial success in the modern world hinges on each parent's ability to roll with the punches and get back to the basics when needed.

This book will not prevent blow-ups from ever happening, but my hope is that it will help minimize the times they do. This book is about creating moments throughout parents' lives to help them remember exactly how they ideally want to parent, regardless of what they might have done just ten minutes before. Remember, we raise families because it is about creating meaning and joy in *our* lives as well as for our children. I want this book to send parents a clear message: Your own happiness should come first, and this ain't something you should apologize for.

Maybe it is better stated this way: It is up to each of us to define our own perfect way of parenting. If perfection even exists for a parent, it surely isn't about being a robot that never makes mistakes. It's about being a human who knows who he/she is in spite of his/her mistakes and works to continually express the best of himself/herself in the world. It is about building a practice of being a healthier and happier person (and parent, and spouse) into our daily lives. The better we do that, the healthier and happier our families are.

Or . . .

Perhaps we dispense of the concept of perfection altogether. Perfect, shmerfect. Because your children are their own people, even a right-feeling decision as a parent can be a potential wrong one because of the way your child might react. So, maybe no go on the perfecto. Instead, let us focus on getting better at calling audibles, being able to change and adjust our tactics in the moment, refusing to get stuck in a certain way, and instead becoming fluid, elastic, versatile, confident, strong.

My wife and I had already been married nearly nine years before we had our first child. Neither she nor I regret waiting that long. In that time, we got to know ourselves and each other better. We worked hard, pursued our passions, and, in some cases, had enough time and space to reassess what our passions actually were. When we finally decided to start a family, we were ready.

My goal with this book is to help parents and parents-to-be of all ages learn or relearn who they are as parents and where their own passions may lie. My belief is that being a successful parent means devoting time to something you are passionate about that is entirely independent of the family.

For those of you who follow me and/or have read my first book, you may not be surprised that I'm venturing into the parenting realm. Or maybe you're wondering why the heck I'm doing this.

Over the years, I have worked with incredible individuals searching for a better way to live their lives. And their lives are entangled with the lives of their partners and children. There is, in fact, no separation, and their desire to live better means an inevitable attention to the family. For them, and for myself, I believe it is time for a philosophy-of-parenting book that is 100 percent happiness focused and has absolutely nothing to do with tools that will turn your child into a musical-poetry-math prodigy. Not to say that a violin-playing, sonnet-writing, square-root-a-calculating virtuoso wouldn't be cool—but only as long as they're happy, right?

Read this book. Take the ideas that work for you, and make them your own. I work to help people become who they choose to be. And that goes for the parents they choose to be, too. Who they truly are, the parents they truly are. Get to know that, and you have a goal and a direction. Get to know that, and you let go of the guilt, the pressure, the stress, the regret. I believe we, as parents, have a goal, and a reason to chase that goal no matter what. The goal? A happy and healthy family life. The most human connection we have, and one that easily gets lost in the daily shuffle of our lives.

One final note: I am in my own practice with this. I have the same struggles, fears, and worries as most parents. I know that some of you reading this do the job of parenting better than I do, while some have a harder time than I with this monumentally difficult task. No matter. I want the ideas in this book to inspire you and possibly change your perspective. I want the practical tools in this book to make your parenting life just a tad easier. Above all, my hope is that this book serves as a reminder of what is more important than jobs, money, and technology.

I wish you all the success in the world. The better you do individually, the better example you set. The better example you set, the better your child does, the better your family does, the better the world does. You win, we all win.

I HAVE THE SAME STRUGGLES, FEARS, AND WORRIES AS MOST PARENTS.

UCTION INTRO
INTRODUCTION
UCTION INTRO
INTRODUCTION
UCTION INTRO

I wanted to write a book that would get you to look at your role as a parent differently than possibly ever before. To understand that to be a successful father, mother, but also a musician, lawyer, mechanic, teacher, takes an ethic of self-care. A focus on you as a human before you as a parent, you as a lawyer, and so on.

Enter *Raising Healthy Parents*.

This is not a conventional parenting book, so keep that in mind as you thumb through these pages. This is, above all, a philosophy book. It's a human-in-the-world book. It's a natural-species-in-an-unnatural-world book. It's a damn-is-it-tough-to-stay-happy-and-healthy-these-days book. It's a we-can-do-this-and-do-it-better book.

I wrote my first book, *Approaching the Natural: A Health Manifesto*, with a similar idea in mind—to cut through the crap and get back to some basic principles about how to live the best lives we can. *Raising Healthy Parents* is that for me, too, but in the context of the family dynamic. It's no small feat to raise a happy and healthy child, much like it's no small feat to maintain a happy and healthy marriage. Yet we embark on the struggle because the benefit so far outweighs the hardship, that it's not even in the same ballpark. We might—in a nice, quiet room, maybe a fire in the fireplace, a cup of hot tea in our hands—tell anyone who asks how having a child is wonderful and fulfilling and brings a daily smile to our faces. We'll tell you how the birth of our child was the most profound, spiritual moment of our lives. We'll tell you we can't even remember how our lives were before we had children. And then . . .

The day hits.

The carpool, the job, the errands, the financial worry, the news, and a bunch of other stuff hitting us, making us vulnerable to anger, irritability, and stress. And then, with all this on our shoulders, we spend time with our partners and children. All that we know about how awesome and fulfilling it is to raise a family gets very quiet. It gets shoved to the back so that we can get to the business of getting through the day.

Result? Decreased health, vibrancy, happiness in the family.

And so . . . a few words on what to expect in this book.

My initial idea for a book about healthy families was a more traditional organized-by-chapter book, but as I began writing, I watched it turn into something else entirely. Fortunately, my publisher and editor were game with the new direction, so here it is.

I've designed the book to be something you can pick up, read a few pages from, and put down so you can get back to your day. Any book, no matter how excellent the information, is useless if it's so boring, dry, and unwieldy that it sits on the shelf . . . I want this book to be fun, even funny at times, but so accessible and easy to read that you can steal a few minutes with it here and there to get some good information and inspiration without worrying that you'll have trouble remembering where you left off. Use it as a tool that might help you reconnect to what you know deep down about yourself and your family.

I have been interested in nutrition and overall healthy living (as you'll read, my philosophy of health encompasses much more than food) for the better part of my life, and this interest certainly preceded any actual work for me in the field. In 1992, as a singer-songwriter and after reading one of the first of many health books, I made a relatively small change in my diet and found myself free of asthma for the first time.

For the next seventeen years, still as a singer-songwriter but as a working actor as well, I read health book after health book, experimenting with diets, fasts, and cleanses. (Someday, when we know each other better, I'll tell you about a wheatgrass cleanse my wife and I did in 1994 and that I'm still traumatized by—suffice it to say, we got to know each other a bit *too* well . . . we don't talk about it.) In 2009, with a healthy-living interest still burning strong, and our twins on the way, I returned to school to formally study nutrition and earn a certification.

You might be wondering why a singer-songwriter-actor would care so much about healthy living . . . because I realized immediately the impact it had on the overall quality of my life. I saw clearly from the beginning that no matter what I pursued, no matter what my interests were, taking care of myself could enable me to *do more*. To be more fulfilled. To have more and greater experiences.

These days, I coach people for a living. I run a wellness center for a living. I write books, record podcasts, create YouTube videos for a living. And still, even with this completely different career in motion, I see that the priority I set years ago of taking care of myself still enables me today to do what I love. I see that no matter what my passions have been, the through line of self-care and health has delivered me the goods.

But far more important than any job or career I've ever had or ever will have, devoting attention to my own health and happiness has paid off big time in my family life, in my ability to parent effectively, and in my ability to have and maintain a successful marriage.

Again, my philosophy of health is a broad-stroke approach, encompassing diet, movement, creativity, socialization, and even pursuits such as journaling and meditation. It is essentially an approach to being happy in our lives using all the areas I just listed as tools.

The argument I make in this book is fairly simple: Being a successful parent means first being a successful human. And being a successful human means being happy, healthy, vibrant, compassionate, creative, and truly alive.

What I've found time and time again in my health-coaching practice is an ethic that, for some reason, has fallen by the wayside: the ethic of self-care. My challenge with many clients is to teach them how to take care of themselves again. Not by shoving broccoli down their throats, but by finally paying real attention to the lives they want to live. Rarely are clients' weight issues actually about food or a lack of basic knowledge about what constitutes healthy eating. Overwhelmingly, they're about not living life on their own terms. Their lives have gotten away from them—they are overstressed, distracted, and fatigued, and not-so-healthy food is just the ticket after a crappy day at work.

My work, often long before any discussion of food, is to help my clients get clear about the life they want to live. What follows at that point is to take steps to live that life more each day. As that life unfolds, healthy changes in eating and exercise come naturally and organically. Unforced, minimally stressful, sustainable, long term.

Thing is? This work applies 100 percent to parents, too.

As a parent of three children (did I mention I have twins?), I understand the inherent difficulty in finding some time for ourselves, much less real, uninterrupted time with our spouses/partners. For me, it is *the* struggle of the modern world, and the inspiration for this book.

So . . .

Two assumptions: 1) You're a parent or parent-to-be, and 2) you're busy.

Raising Healthy Parents is a book written and organized specifically to cater to those two assumptions. If you happen to be a nonparent with a ton of time on your hands, well, I'm at a loss as to why you'd read this book—but, hey, who am I to judge?

I've split the book into two main sections: Philosophy and Reality.

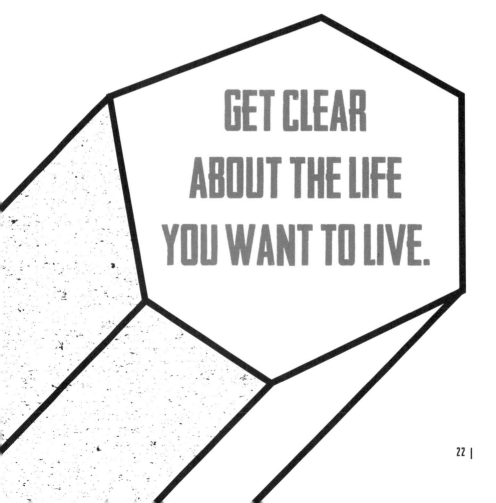

GET CLEAR
ABOUT THE LIFE
YOU WANT TO LIVE.

PHILOSOPHY FIRST

W hy philosophy first? Because before you get into the nitty-gritty of eating and exercise, I want you to have the context within which these changes will occur. For me, it is about the ideas first. When the ideas and the overall philosophy are clear, the stage is set for long-term change. The ideas are the foundation and the grounding force, and what keeps us from bouncing around from plan to plan, from diet to diet, from strategy to strategy, without devoting enough time to any one thing to allow it to fully take effect.

In this section, I introduce you to the ideas that form the basis of my overall Small Steps approach to long-term, truly sustainable change. You'll ask yourself the big questions, like what kind of parent you want to be and what being an ideal parent even means to you.

Also in this section, I address what I consider to be the ethic of healthy parenting. For me, this is an ethical issue because it is about how we treat both ourselves and our families. About kindness and compassion and, in a very real sense, having the strength to do the right thing.

You will read about the state of the modern world, and the struggle inherent in it. I never underestimate the amount of work it takes for each of us to eke out a healthy life on an individual level, much less the additional effort to achieve this outcome for our families.

Integral to my overall message is an acceptance of struggle, and acceptance that it is precisely the hard work of this process that delivers us the happiness we desire. *Raising Healthy Parents* is not about removing the struggle, but rather about embracing it—making success a real possibility because we're more aware than ever before of the payoff . . .

By the end of the first section, you will have a clear picture of what being a successful human being means to you. What being a successful parent means to you. What a thriving family looks like to you. At that point, you will be ready for the section that follows . . .

REALITY SETS IN

In the Reality section, I answer this question: "Fine, but what do I actually do, like, today?"

This section is where I put the ideas into action. I have had great success with my unique Small Steps approach, and it is in this section that you'll learn the ins and outs of how to proceed. I will show you that no matter how busy you are, no matter what the day-to-day logistics of your life are (soccer, carpool, job, grocery shopping, etc.), you can, via Small Steps, build in actual quality time for yourself. Just the time you need to have the strength and focus to execute the style of parenting and health you came to know while reading the Philosophy section.

In this section I apply my Small Steps approach to all the elements that, when in place, lead to increased health and happiness: food, movement, and even nonphysical exercise (what I call mental nutrition). All this to help you steer the ship (read: family) to healthier/ happier waters. Understand that all these elements are hard enough for adults to implement for themselves—adding children into the mix makes it all that much more of a challenge.

Fear not.

My Small Steps approach is the perfect system to transition not only you but also your children without major upset or familial stress.

Last, in the Reality section, I've included some of my favorite, yet easiest, recipes. But not many. I explain this in detail later, but short story is that I've found most parents want to minimize the time they spend shopping, prepping, and cooking. Homing in on a select number of dishes in lieu of time spent on weekly meal planning with a ton of variety/changes makes this possible.

And last but not least . . .

A NOTE ON RESEARCH

While I draw on research for *Raising Healthy Parents,* I know that for every research-based point I make in the following pages, readers could find ten studies disproving each point. It is very similar to my work as a health coach and certified nutritionist. Both in the parenting and nutritional landscapes, there are a mind-boggling number of opposing opinions.

With more than enough studies, books, and research to make our heads spin, what is to be done?

Other than my old standby of, "Well, just take my frickin' word for it," I believe in most cases—including nutrition and happy families—a return to some common sense is in order. Nutritionally, that means appealing to our physical design and evolution and then trying to apply that knowledge to the world we live in today. Family-wise, I also believe it is simpler than we think. Understanding our evolution as a tribal species and keeping a firm and steady gaze on what the nature of parenting actually is, we stay focused on what is, at its most basic level, our job as parents: to teach our children the ways of the world and impart enough wisdom, knowledge, and confidence to empower them to forge their own happy, fulfilling lives. The more often we remember this, the better our chances of success.

This is easier said than done, of course . . .

Hence this book that I am so passionate and excited about. Here goes . . .

PHILO
SOPHY
PHILO
SOPHY

SOPHY

PHILOS

SOPHY

PHILOS

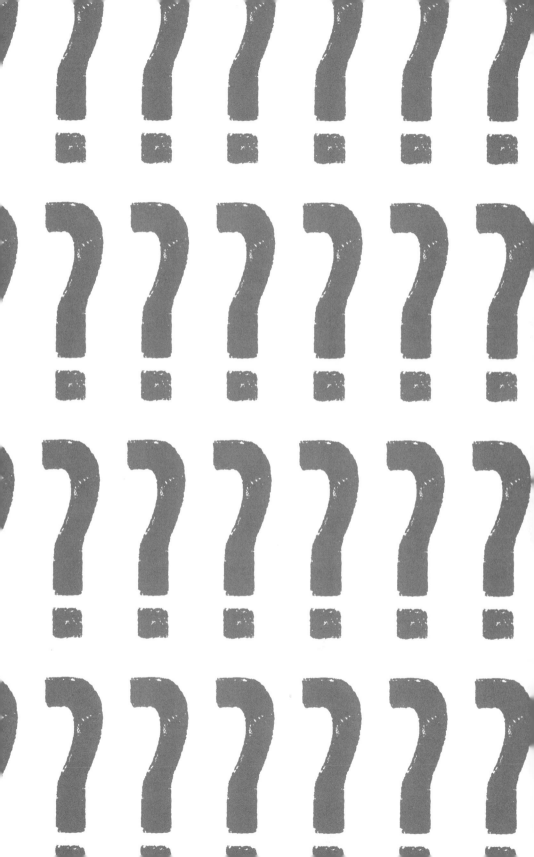

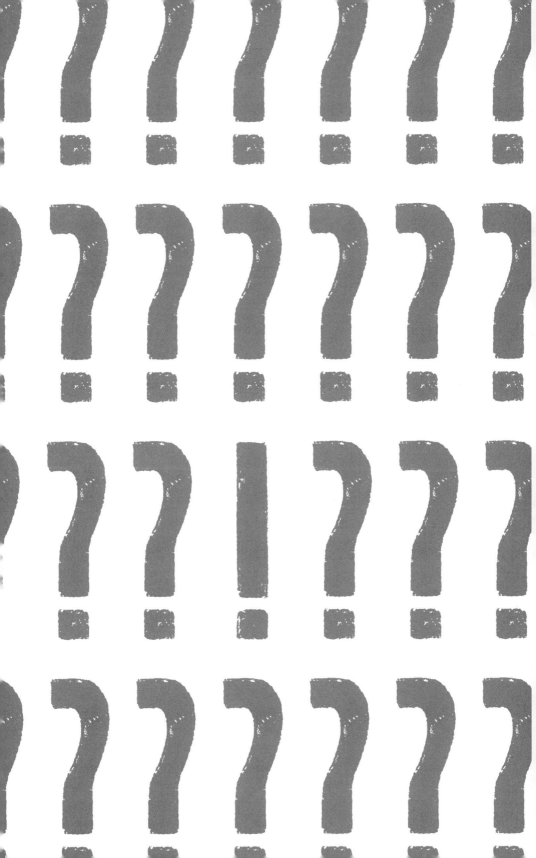

EVERYTHING WILL BECOME APPARENT

IT'S ALL ABOUT YOU

For a moment, let's set aside all the ways we differentiate and categorize ourselves—culture, economics, race, religion, location. The fact is, beneath (or perhaps, above?) all of this are substantially more similarities than differences. The human body is designed to strive for the best health it can achieve. It works as hard as it can no matter what the environment or circumstance. It is always attempting to detox, fight infection, repair, digest, and clean out. In other words, the trillions of things going on in your body as you read this aren't happening to shuttle you more quickly to the Great Beyond. They're to keep you alive as long as possible. The human mind? Same deal. We (you know, the personalities of us) are designed to be on the lookout for more happiness and joy—to minimize mental (emotional/psychological) stress in our lives. This is simply what humans do.

Let's make this the starting point, before everything else to come. Happiness, low stress, low conflict, more fun. Ever met anyone who doesn't want those things? Probably not. Differences among humans come from the ways in which we attempt to achieve them. Self-help books, diet books, exercise DVDs, technology, meditation tapes? All are designed to get us "there" as fast as possible and with minimal perceived effort. Junk food, drugs, alcohol, movies, television? Again, all designed for maximum pleasure with minimal effort. Only one problem: True health and happiness, the kinds that are real and long lasting, don't come easily or quickly. They come from thought and attention, with a heaping scoop of awareness and struggle thrown in.

Notice how I haven't mentioned the word *parent*, nor even a word that rhymes with *parent*? That's because we're not there yet. Stick with me.

Everything will become *apparent* . . .

Nailed it.

Parenting (there, I said it) is about the parent. Yes, books about how to raise, develop, deal with, and communicate with your child line the virtual and physical shelves. How to change your child's behavior, relate to your child, make his/her brain run like a Ferrari. All great stuff, but not my focus. My focus is where I believe 99 percent of the focus should be—on you. Yes, you. The parent. Difficult as it may be, while you read this book, try your best to *not* think about your child or your relationship with your child. Think about you. Your life. Your happiness. Your (forgotten?) dreams and passions. All those amazing child-rearing books have their place, but philosophical questions and considerations come first.

That human beings, parents and nonparents alike, are wired to minimize stress and energy expenditure is fantastic, but that puts us in a pickle in the modern world when it comes to raising and maintaining a healthy family. We're surrounded by an unprecedented amount of technology designed for one thing and one thing only: to make things easier for us, not harder. The human brain is unparalleled in its ability to craft solutions to perceived challenges. Take, for example, the massive problem we faced in the middle of the twentieth century when we were forced to walk sometimes up to ten feet to the television to change a channel. Solution? The invention of the remote control. Problem solved and just in time. One less reason to move our bodies. Now, how we access information, travel, communicate, and even eat has gotten faster and more efficient, but at the same time, these technologies actually move us further from the comparatively simple physical and mental needs of the human animal. Almost daily we figure out new ways to achieve more with less effort—to change the channel without having to get up . . . and yet, just because we can figure out solutions doesn't always mean we should.

The pickle for the human race? The very "solutions" designed to decrease stress aren't making us healthier, happier, or less frickin' stressed.

The pickle for parents? To minimize familial stress on a given day or moment, we will make decisions that do not serve our family's long-term health and happiness. Our intense need for peace can easily outweigh more difficult, yet more valuable, actions. Evidence of this often manifests in the way we feed our children. The brilliant technology of fast food means a cheap, convenient, and enjoyable meal. It's the perfect way to keep our children momentarily happy and fed, while virtually eliminating the struggle that comes with feeding our children healthy food—the struggle of shopping, prepping, cooking, cleaning, not to mention any actual battles over the food itself. Is it any wonder that caring, tired, and stressed parents will opt for a quick fix in order to avoid the battle?

Similarly, putting our children in front of a movie or iPad at the dinner table at the end of the day, while an easy way to attain the much-needed end-of-day quiet, does not reap the long-term benefits of conversation, human interaction, and familial intimacy. Short-term win, long-term loss.

So, does the problem of our children's increasingly poor health come from the fact that we don't *know* that junk food is bad for our children, and that putting them in front of a screen all the time isn't the best thing ever? Of course not. We know. But . . . we're frickin' tired, and we need relief.

As a health coach/nutritionist, I work with people who come to me for weight loss and/or to learn how to eat better. But every single one has a pretty darn good idea about what healthy eating looks like. Rarely is it an issue about not knowing. In the early days of my practice, I made the mistake of focusing solely on food—eat this, this, and this, and by gum, you'll lose the weight. But I soon came to realize it wasn't really about the food. I realized that it was the state of the person and how she/he related to food. If I could coach them in ways that would minimize the nonfood stress of their lives, they wouldn't need the Ben and Jerry's as much. A definite aha! moment for me.

But I digress.

Parenting? Same deal. The information out there about child development, parenting styles, and parent-to-child communication is real and valid. But when push comes to shove, it's more complicated than saying, "Hey, feed your child green beans" or "Talk to your child at the dinner table." Because most of us already have a basic idea of what is good for our kids, and we desperately want to put our knowledge into practice. So, we tell ourselves, "All right, let's get this done!" and "Game on." I'm paraphrasing, of course. But the gist is that we make big plans and our intention is to kick into gear big-time.

Well, except . . .

On days where we have to, you know, get all the crap done that we have to deal with just to keep the ship moving—commutes, jobs, carpools, banking, taxes, bills, dental appointments, keeping in touch with family/friends, laundry, and oh, so much more. Prepare and feed my kids a healthy meal? Great idea. I'll start it tomorrow when I'm not exhausted, rushing home from work, and trying to get them to bed at a decent hour. Yes, tomorrow. There's always tomorrow.

Or . . .

I learn how to take care of myself better. Learn how to find time throughout my day to recharge, reconnect, reground so that . . . wait for it . . . I'm not so exhausted at the end of the day. So I don't walk in the door irritable, fatigued, and stressed. So I have the strength and fortitude to put some healthy food on the table and have a relaxed chat with Joyce, Jan, and/or Franklin.

Why and/or? Please . . . you know how Franklin can be.

A BRAND-NEW PARENT (AGAIN)

The periodic shifts in parenting approaches are eerily similar to the way fad diets come and go. From cry-it-out to co-parenting, from hands-off to helicopter. Most trends are backed by studies, but have you ever asked yourself, "If they're all backed by studies, how can there be two completely conflicting approaches?" The victims of these often-wide swings in parenting approaches (and healthy-eating approaches, for that matter) are the parents themselves, who get bounced around like a pinball. Not only do most parents not have the time to actually read the supporting studies, we don't even have the time to read the books based on the studies. At best, we grab the headlines, book titles, or blog posts, or the cute and tidy little CNN articles. (They're sensational!!!)

My message? Avoid falling prey to these shifts by doing these two things:

1. Know who you are as a parent.
2. Be hyperaware that you *ARE* a parent.

I'll explain and clarify both soon . . . in the meantime:

Let's start at the very beginning. If you're already a parent, remember for a moment how you felt just before the birth of your first child. If you're a parent-to-be or planning on having a child at some point, you're in it, so just be in it. In what? In the fear, the not-knowing, the adventure, the anxiety, the excitement. So many feelings swirling around your brain all at once for one of the most natural of human experiences.

And yet, when you really think about it, for today's human animal, it's a decidedly unnatural event. Ever seen an animal give birth? Most have a look on their face (yes, I'm projecting) of, "Yeah, this is what I'm doing right now. It's just something I *do*." Not humans. We have birth plans, lactation coaches, doulas, midwives, hospitals, medications, not to mention the sci-fi-like metal tools used to extract a little alien out of our bodies (by *our*, I mean not mine or any other man's, but you have to admit that most men are super good at standing in the vicinity). There is a disconnect right from the get-go. In theory, for men and women, this should be like it is for other animals. Just something we do and keep doing, with little fanfare. But it's just not.

We've got amazing, creative brains, intricate language, and yet are so much in the dark when it comes to first giving birth and then parenting. Makes sense when you think about it—as our world becomes more complicated and unnatural, parenting and childbirth become more complicated and unnatural as well. It is no longer about children learning the basic, natural survival skills (find food, find shelter, escape from predators), because they don't live in nature. Today, we have to teach our children the modern version of survival skills—study hard in school; get a job; know the difference between healthy and unhealthy food; don't get bullied or be a bully; and know how to dress, pay taxes, drive a car, and a thousand other intricacies that muddle our brains. In other words, it's no longer, "Hey, this thing on the ground? You can eat it." Rather, it's, "Hey, go to school, get a job, earn a paycheck, take that paycheck to the bank and deposit it, head to the market, use your money to buy and eat *these* foods most of the time, and not *these* foods that often, but either way, take the food you buy home, do stuff to it, and then, only then, eat it. Oh, wait, you gotta do the dishes after that." Wow, I just got runner's high from writing all that.

Point is, when we become/became a parent, we become/became a teacher with a job description the size of *War and Peace*. The BIG, capitalized question is this: WHAT KIND OF TEACHER DO YOU WANT TO BE?

Here's where I ask you to humor me for a moment. Indulge me in a little, well, hippie-dippy, new-agey, touchy-feely exercise. Get over it. Work with me here. Just frickin' do what I'm asking you to do, for the love of all that's holy.

This exercise is the cornerstone of this entire book and my entire Small Steps coaching approach. It's the backbone of all the practical tools of this book's second half. It works. After you complete the exercise, I'll tell you why. Here goes:

THE PARENT WE ACTUALLY ARE

Instructions: If you were the bestest, most awesome parent in the world, what would that look like? Don't compare yourself to anyone else or any other family. Think about just you, your family, what you'd be doing, and how you'd be acting if you were doing the best parenting job you possibly could.

This is what I want you to describe in the section that follows, *but* . . . write it as if it's already happening. If you're not yet a parent, just pretend you have a child already. If you already have children, disregard every single thing you've done as a parent up to now. Pretend you've lost your memory completely, but I'm telling you that you are the model parent, and, knowing that, write down what you do as this parent. I have provided an example to give you an idea, *but* it's just an example and may not be at all what you write. Get as specific as you can. Take a few minutes here and really give it some thought. Before you write a single word, really picture yourself as this parent. One more time: Write all your descriptions as if they're happening now. Not "I eventually will do this," but rather "I do this." Give it the old college try and know that you can always change and update this exercise.

A PERSONAL EXAMPLE

I am calm most of the time. Even if I have a stressful day at work, I'm able to "leave it at the office" and be positive and fun at home. I don't expect to never get angry or lose my temper, but it doesn't happen often. If I do get angry, I quickly catch myself. I have no problem acknowledging and apologizing when I make mistakes. I am supportive of my children and wife. I want my children to be happy and strong. I understand that they rely on me to be their parent and guide and that this comes way before being their friend. My spouse and I are a united front, always backing each other up when it comes to the rules and expectations of the household.

Okay, that's my example. This exercise might feel a little uncomfortable to write, but I urge you to push through it no matter how foreign or weird what you write seems. Create a picture in your head and write what you see.

Ready, set, go:

_____

_____

_____

_____

_____

_____

_____

_____

_____

Philosophy

_____
_____
_____
_____
_____
_____
_____
_____
_____
_____
_____
_____
_____
_____
_____
_____
_____
_____
_____
_____
_____
_____
_____
_____

How did that feel? Inauthentic? Like a romp through fantasy land? As you wrote it, did you hear a voice in your head saying, "This is crap—you don't look remotely like the person you just described"? Or were there some parts of what you wrote that are pretty fair representations of how you already behave as a parent? Or, are you exactly the parent you described in the exercise?

I argue that the parent you described above is the true you. Those actions and character traits are what you hold as your own values, standards, and ideals. They define you. You are, in your head, the adult you just described. (If you're a child reading this, then . . . seriously? Go play a video game. Preferably one that looks as if you're playing outside.)

Here's what'll twist your noodle: It is 100 percent irrelevant how you've actually *been* as a parent up to this point. I'll explain what I mean by relating it to what I do in my Small Steps coaching practice . . .

At the very beginning of my work with any client, I have them do a task similar to the one above (essentially, the nonparenting version—health themed), which I brilliantly and imaginatively call "The First Task." In this task, some will write, "I am at, and maintain, a healthy weight," even though they are actually overweight. Some will write, "I do not overeat," despite the fact that they are self-described bingers. The task becomes the basis for all the work we do together, since, by writing their ideal, they are clearly laying out their goals regarding their own health and happiness. Often, during our work together, I'll ask, "What would be the first task *you* do in this situation?" The task serves as an excellent reference during times of indecision and allows my clients to become clearer than ever before about who they are and what they stand for.

Simply stated, it's damn nice to be clear about that so you have something to work toward.

The work it takes to become (and stay) the best parent you can be isn't about becoming a *different* parent; it's about starting to act more like the one you are. It just may be that in some areas, the way you've been acting is at odds with how you'd *rather* be acting . . .

If reading what you wrote makes you feel bad about how you've actually been parenting, ask yourself why. Actually, don't bother asking, because I'm telling you: How you've been parenting simply isn't a good representation of the real you. The real you is the person you described in the writing. This book is about getting that person off the page and into the real world more and more each day. No more beating yourself up—it's a colossal waste of time. Enough already. It's time to finally be *you*. It's time to create a lifelong practice whereby you act a little more like that parent on the page each day.

Having a child and guiding your child makes you a parent. But the ability to be an effective, positive force in your child's life has nothing to do with your child. It has to do with the *you* in the relationship. Unfortunately, most of us don't devote nearly enough time to the question of what kind of parent we actually want to be. We just go from parenting moment to parenting moment, either judging ourselves along the way or figuring out how to compartmentalize that judgment so we don't feel crappy about the job we are doing.

Until we find out what the picture of our ideal parent looks like, how we parent is most likely either eerily similar to how we were parented or eerily opposite to how we were parented. In contrast, the above exercise identifies *our* approach and gives us something to work toward. When we have a firm knowledge of our approach, when we become fatigued, irritable, stressed, and lost, we at least have a place to come home to. A place where we can check in with the parent we actually are and refocus our efforts for the future.

HEY, PAST, CAN YOU HANG OUT FOR ONE MORE SEC BEFORE YOU GO?

Allow me a little bit o' trite: We can't change the past. We can wallow in it, regret it, get pissed about it, spend a whole bunch of time analyzing it, but we can't change the damn thing. At the same time, while it's a neat idea to just "Let it go, man," I think we'd be losing out on an excellent opportunity for growth and knowledge by giving the past a little look-see before sending it on its way.

My approach is definitely forward thinking. You're looking to become a better parent in your future. But taking a moment to see how you've been acting, then comparing that with what you now know about yourself (because of the previous task), is not only great to know but will also make you a little more self-aware next time around. Perhaps you'll catch yourself a little quicker when you walk in the door in an irritable mood. But isn't it nice to look at the way you've been walking in the door, recognize that behavior as something you are not, then become even more clear about who you are in hopes that you'll get a handle on it over time? I agree. It is nice.

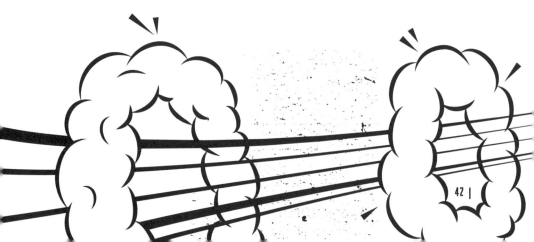

MAKE THE TRADE

I'm assuming that you're reading this book either because you want to improve the health and happiness of your family or you want to learn a minimally stressful way to maintain it. Either way, the overall goal is simple: It'd be great to have a good life. I call this the "umbrella goal" because it covers all the particular actions we may take to achieve and/ or maintain a happy family, such as the food our families eat, the quality of time our families spend together, etc. All roads point to making our existence on this earth as individuals and families as good as possible. Sound trite? Oversimplified? Not possible, since our goal really is this simple. Let's cut the crap for a moment, put down the gargantuan stack of books showing us how to raise the next Einstein by fusing our child's right and left brains or how we can raise the next Mozart by wrapping a belt around a pregnant belly that plays frickin' Mozart (And isn't this cheating? I mean, the kid's gonna be born already knowing all the songs), and remember what we're actually shooting for when we do these things. If we can't look beyond the Mozart belt or the Einstein-making nutty nut nut, our parenting worlds become very narrowed. We become hyperfocused on our child's intelligence and musical talent and forget to ask whether our child is happy or, just as important, whether we are happy.

By making our family's happiness the goal, with health an absolutely essential part of this goal, we get past the perceptions of restriction that hover over individual healthy actions. Food is a perfect example of where this perception comes into play. Many parents want their children to eat healthier food but feel it would be restrictive to not let their kids eat whatever they feel like or to not let them make their own decisions about food. But think about it this way: If feeding your child a technically more restrictive diet (e.g., by perhaps restricting the amount of junk food at home) helps your child think more clearly, feel better, be more active, be happier, be more focused in school, then how restrictive is your choice, really?

I call it "making the trade," which is a way to think about the changes you make for yourself and your family. You trade an action in one narrow, specific area of your life in exchange for an overall happier, joyful life. Good trade.

In 1992, after a lifetime of asthma, I read *Fit for Life* and decided to give up dairy (milk, cheese, yogurt). Within a month, my asthma was gone, and I was an "inhaler-packin' guy" no longer. I had graduated from college the year before and was pursuing a career as a singer-songwriter. Singer . . . get it? Asthma and singing don't mix. Sure, I've heard 14,327 times (literally), "I could never give up cheese," but when I did, my quality of life immediately shot up. Strictly speaking, I did restrict my diet. I had been eating dairy, and I was now cutting it out completely. But my focus was on how much better I felt, how much less effort it took to sing. Fact is, I could have continued to eat dairy, but I chose not to. And I've stuck to it—there's no tension around that decision, because I know what it has brought me.

Decide to improve your family's diet? Make the "rules" of healthy eating secondary to the "why." Rules alone will land you and your family in a restrictive cloud of misery and stress. Remember the "why," and you'll be fine with a little food restriction because you know that overall this makes for greater happiness. Great trade.

Other trades? Trade an earlier bedtime for a well-rested, happier, less-stressed, better-behaved child. Trade less television for a well-read, more imaginative, more creative child.

Makes the parenting required to pull these trades off completely worth the struggle. Remember in the intro, when I wrote about how nothing worthwhile in the world comes without struggle? This is what I'm talking about. And . . . someone has to be prepared for this struggle so they can meet it with strength, vitality, and happiness. Someone has to be focused enough, strong enough to make the trade. That someone? No, but good guess. Answer? You. You, and only you.

The fact is that for any change you make on your family's behalf to be meaningful, it's got to be long term and sustainable. (Not hippie "sustainable." The actual sustainable—like, you can keep going with it.) You can't expect a week of healthy eating to do much more than cause you a world of hassle. Real results come with time and effort, and we have to be in the right frame of mind to make this happen for our families. That means keeping an eye on the ball as much as possible so that any worries about restriction are put where they belong. In the trash, or the dustbin, as the Brits call it.

Often, I'll advise clients *not* to change a thing about the food they eat until they become very clear about their own umbrella goals, which are, trust me, way bigger than a number on a scale or a leaf of kale. I want their heads in the umbrella goal long before they add a stalk of celery to whatever else they're eating for dinner. I want them to notice the trade they're making long before they make real-life changes like minimizing fast food. When they're hyperaware of the trade, the chances of continuing the healthier habit go through the roof.

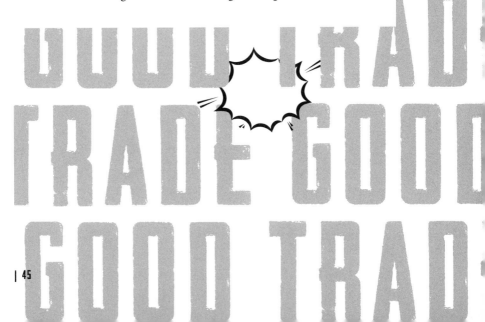

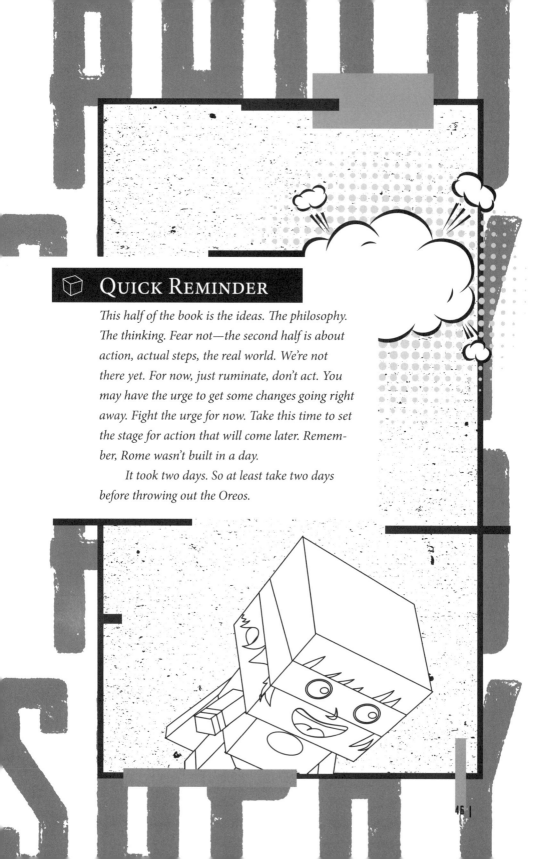

📦 QUICK REMINDER

This half of the book is the ideas. The philosophy. The thinking. Fear not—the second half is about action, actual steps, the real world. We're not there yet. For now, just ruminate, don't act. You may have the urge to get some changes going right away. Fight the urge for now. Take this time to set the stage for action that will come later. Remember, Rome wasn't built in a day.

It took two days. So at least take two days before throwing out the Oreos.

MOTT

Your MOTT, your family's MOTT. It's the determining factor of your success in both the health and happiness realms. What is a MOTT? Most. Of. The. Time.

Here's the deal. It's what you do most of the time that sets your level of health and happiness. Like right now. Right now, how happy you are as a family is based on how you and your children communicate most of the time, how you all eat most of the time, how you all move your bodies most of the time, how you all behave around friends and extended family most of the time.

Here is why I'm MOTT's biggest fan: Because it is completely not about an *all* of the time. It's about "most." It's human, real, doable.

Thinking in MOTT terms means not sweating the one-offs.

Think you should be able to pull off a no-mistake, 100-percent-perfection existence, and you're setting yourself up for failure. Period.

Nobody, and I mean nobody, likes making a mistake. And where children are affected, mistakes kick up to a whole new level. Making a parenting mistake is a very different animal than forgetting to pay the phone bill.

In the back of a parent's mind is a fear that even a single mistake will land our child in therapy years later.

Child to therapist: "This one time my dad forgot to pay the phone bill, and I couldn't call my friend, and I see now that my inability to hold down a job or a healthy relationship stems from that one unpaid bill."

Luckily, in most cases, here-and-there screw-ups don't add up to much. But with MOTT, it's not about the one-offs.

The concept of MOTT even applies to one's diet. The health of your diet is determined by what you eat most of the time. If you eat junk food and take-out most of the time, with a salad thrown in once a week, your

MOTT ain't the salad. It's the junk food and take-out, and the health of your body will likely reflect that (unless you're some sort of freak who runs super well on fries). The salad doesn't play a big enough role in your movie to even get an end credit. But if your MOTT is healthy food, with a fast food meal thrown in now and then, the opposite is true. Your MOTT is healthy food, and the one fast food meal ain't gonna break the bank. By the way, you'll learn everything you need to know about nutrition for you and your family in the Reality section, so fear not, and don't frickin' skip ahead. We're not there yet.

Here's where it gets even more interesting. The MOTT concept goes for the mind, too. For your happiness. Does your MOTT with your spouse or partner consist of open, respectful communication with an argument once in a while, or of arguments most of the time, with a bouquet of flowers thrown in on Valentine's Day? Do the math. The one-offs don't tip the scales or break the bank. They do neither, because they're not significant enough to make any difference.

Here are the reasons I wish everyone would embrace MOTT:

1. You don't beat yourself up over a once-in-a-while mistake if it's not your MOTT.
2. If you increase the quality of your food MOTT, you will actually enjoy the special, less-healthy meals even more. As in, you improve the quality of food you eat most of the time, and you're feeling and looking pretty darn good. At that point, you care a lot less about what you might eat while traveling or at a party. You've got a kick-ass MOTT as your foundation. Because I eat really well most of the time, the seven-layer Taco Bell burrito (no cheese, no sour cream) is a guilt-free indulgence. On the other hand, if said brilliantly crafted burrito were my MOTT, I'd very soon enjoy it a lot less. Oh, and I wouldn't be nearly as healthy or happy . . .

3. The more you think in terms of your MOTT, you quickly notice, without the always charming and supportive inner critic, when your MOTT needs a little tweaking. All the time you previously wasted feeling bad about periodic flubs is now devoted to bringing up your MOTT. Your focus is on the improvement—on what you are doing way more than what you're not doing.

4. You get perspective. You don't think your family is going to hell in a handbasket just because you got into a fight with your daughter over some dirty dishes. And you can actually communicate this to your daughter when the argument is over—i.e., communicate the perspective itself (e.g., "Look, this is just one argument, and you're doing really well overall. I just need you to help out more in this one area.")

5. Because your focus is on your MOTT and not the one-offs, you begin to think in terms of patterns. It's the difference between a businessperson who freaks out and makes sweeping changes because of a single bad review versus the person who realizes you can't please everyone and, as long as *most* of the reviews are good, then something's obviously working. Same for your life—thinking in terms of your MOTT means you also quickly notice when the MOTT itself needs a little tune-up . . .

NOT EVERYTHING
IN MODERATION

Don't mistake MOTT for everyone's favorite go-to: Everything in moderation.

I've come to loathe "Everything in moderation" like I've come to loathe the word *should*. Big pet peeve of mine. The cleverest then clarify: Everything in moderation, *even* moderation. Hmmm. My brain hurts trying to wrap it around that nonsense. Looks great on a poster, but we're trying to build and maintain a family full of grounded, happy, healthy people.

So what's my beef with "Everything in moderation"?

Fact is, some things simply aren't okay in moderation. Cheating, stealing, hurting animals and people are not okay, not even just a little bit, and definitely not in moderation. These principles are ethical, they're philosophical, and they're the values we hold whether we've consciously decided to hold them or not.

And yet, "Everything in moderation" is used as a cop-out. A self-issued license to lower your own bar. To not at least strive for greatness, knowing mistakes will be made no matter what. To settle for less than what you know you want to achieve in your life. Don't fall into that trap. Your MOTT isn't that. It isn't about convincing yourself that it is okay to do something you're not okay doing. It's a focus on what you're doing over what you're not doing. It's recognizing what is actually affecting your overall happiness and putting your energy there when you want to improve your life. Your MOTT lives in the food, exercise, and lifestyle realms. In the right/wrong of personal ethics, know the things you're *never* ever okay doing. As it should be.

Know what you stand for, and try to remain standing more often than not. Living by your principles feels good. Let's face it. It feels powerful, strong, energetic. Not treating yourself badly over a minor one-off mistake is a principle of self-care. Living by the MOTT is a principle of self-care. Just the ticket to make yourself a happier, healthier parent. You, your partner/spouse, and your children are too important to either get hung up on absolute perfection or to lower your own expectations with "everything in moderation."

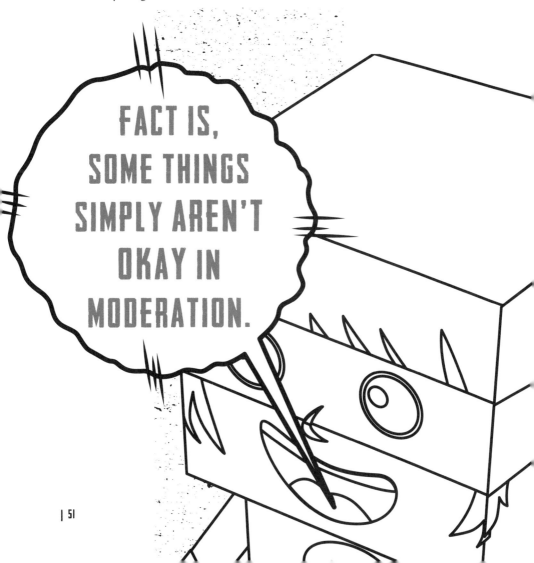

WITH FRIENDS LIKE THESE . . .

Your children are not your friends. You can be friendly with them and have a super-close relationship where you share like friends. But your children are not your friends. One more time to hammer it home: Your children are NOT your friends. Thank goodness for all-caps, because clearly I've made my point.

Whether you like it or not, to our children we are their parents and always will be. From their very first moments on the earth, children look to us for security, guidance, acceptance, support, and love. We succeed when we're both able to and actually do provide all those things. Not one, not two, not three, but all those things. Being your child's friend isn't on that list. And, yes, I made up the list, but it's not on there, so there. And think for a few moments about what I wrote a mere three sentences ago: *able to* and *actually do* provide. To put it another way . . . if you have the ability to be there for your children in these ways and choose not to? Fail. Likewise, if you aren't in a good enough place in your own life to be able to provide your child with necessary guidance, security, etc.? Fail. You can't fake it. Children see right through a checked-out, disconnected parent who feigns support and love. For success (again, most of the time), you've got to be willing *and* able.

We simply cannot parent effectively if we're afraid we won't be liked for some decision we make. We can't sell out our values (take a moment to reread, yet again, the task you completed page 38—those are your values) for the sake of being our kid's buddy. When did we decide it's okay not to parent our kids? When did we decide it's fine to let our kids be loud and run around a restaurant? When did we decide it's cool to let our kids eat whatever they want, watch whatever they want, behave however they want? When did we decide to remove ourselves from the equation?

What happens when we attempt friendship with our children? We behave the way we do with our actual friends. Works great in the friend realm, but not when it comes to our children. What happens is that we let our children make their own choices in the healthy-living arena that they're simply not prepared to make. Why? Because we do that with our friends. We don't tell our friends what they can and can't eat. We don't shop/cook/order for them. They're their own people. So they make their own choices.

Children, on the other hand, while having their own feelings and thoughts, rely on us to help them grow into their own people. I heard a parent say once (in all seriousness), "My child just likes Chicken McNuggets," as if the parent had nothing to do with driving the child, placing the order, and paying, for crying out loud. Of course the child likes McNuggets. They're designed to be liked by children (and adults, of course). More on this later in the book, but it is up to us to make unpopular decisions like, "We don't eat that crap."

Remember that we are animals. Ever read George Orwell's *Animal Farm*? Animals dressing up like people? Yeah, that's us, too. We're animals who don't want to think of ourselves as animals. What this means for us in today's very unnatural/unwild world is that the human animal is up against a whole host of obstacles (those tasty McNuggets are just the tip of the iceberg) that make it very hard for us to achieve any significant level of health and happiness. Now, put a child in this world—see how poorly equipped this little, inexperienced animal is in trying to wade through all this madness?

I've heard so many parents say they "empower" their children to make their own choices about food. Trust me, you're not *empowering* them to do anything. You're essentially letting them loose in the wild and giving them a best-wishes slap on the back. The modern world is a dangerous place if you consider the hidden dangers, physically and psychologically, of junk food, drugs, violent video games, and more. Sure, we're not getting chased by actual lions, but we *are* getting chased by companies trying to ensnare us into habits that will affect our lives and the lives of our children for the worse. Letting your children go unprotected into the wilds of the modern world is simply not fair to them or to you. They lack the necessary skills, and if we don't teach them those skills, they'll eventually become adults who lack them.

Not to get all science-y, but the frontal cortex, the part of the brain that enables us (parents/adults) to make choices that might be different from how we feel in the moment (e.g., I *feel* like having Chicken McNuggets, but I *know* they're not good for me and that I'll regret it if I eat them) takes about twenty-five years to mature. Twenty-five years. To expect a child of eight or sixteen to make the same kind of decision while flying solo is simply unfair. Manufactured food and entertainment is designed to set everyone's heads on fire. If we have a tough time keeping our own urges at bay, imagine how hard it is for your child.

Don't justify putting your children in the position of making a choice between healthy food and junk food or between playing outside and playing a video game on the couch by saying you respect their right to choose what's best for them. Until they're adults, you're in charge of teaching them what's best. They need you to step in and say, "Not this time. Another time, perhaps." They need you to make the rules for them until they can make their own rules, until they become mature enough to ideally make choices that are independent of addiction and temptation. In the meantime, they're looking for you to go to bat for them. They expect you to know and want what's best for them.

Good parenting doesn't make you super popular. But protecting them until they are able to protect themselves will make you a kick-ass parent and will earn their respect. It just makes for a rough day now and then.

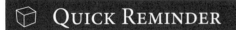

QUICK REMINDER

Don't forget your MOTT. For instance, if you and your family are eating healthy most of the time, are you going to sweat a little junk food now and then? If you allow it, it's still your rule and your choice—not you giving up or giving in.

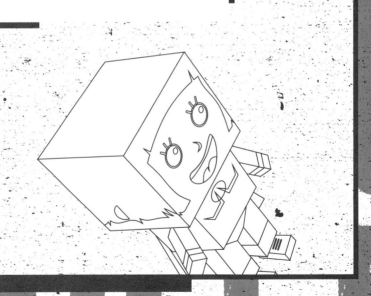

WAIT, *I'M* THE ADULT IN THE ROOM?

Some (my wife) might say I'm emotionally closer to sixteen than I am to forty-eight. Or perhaps that's my level of humor. Either way, I don't feel (and definitely sometimes don't act) like my age. That goes for mind and body.

But . . . there are times when I have to step up and be the frickin' adult. It actually feels very foreign sometimes, as if I'm watching myself playing the part of the adult. Like I'm doing the things that an adult does. One of the tricks to being a successful parent is knowing full well those times when adult-like behavior is essential and those times that it's okay and even good to behave like a kid. Our children can keep us young in our minds and bodies, but . . . best to know when the adult should be front and center. Last thing you want is to end up like Matthew McConaughey's character in *Dazed and Confused*.

My wife and I still have the "Man, this feels so out of place" moments when we're parenting. We both feel like children trapped in adult bodies, and we're just trying to do the best we can. And, to be clear, I think this is a good thing. Feeling and "being" young makes for a fun, exciting, vigorous life, but let's face it—our kids are often looking around for the adult in the room.

It doesn't work at all if we're standing beside them looking, too— wait, *I'm* the adult in the room?

ME, OR NOT ME? THAT IS THE (ONLY) QUESTION

Children are going to kick our asses from time to time. This we know. My hope is that you'll fret less about this once the idea of MOTT sinks in and you've put the concept of the perfect parent right on the ol' trash heap. With that said, I would like to propose a life you could live whereby you could probably minimize getting your ass handed to you. Trust me—as you'll see, it is a completely attainable life for most of us, so if you can make the following a reality, I highly suggest it. (And, if the following is already your life, really no need to finish this book.)

Here goes:

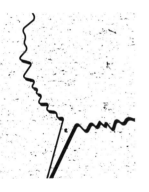

You have someone who cooks for you, cleans for you, drives you everywhere, shops for you, is an on-site marriage counselor, takes the trash out, does the laundry, carpools, tells you every five minutes that you're giving it the ol' college try and doing great, doles out massages as needed—oh, and provides you with a ton of money while making sure you're tucked in at a reasonable hour and woken up each morning to classical music.

Or, if the above is just a smidge tough for you to pull off, then understand this:

Our lives get the best of us from time to time and cause us to behave in not-so-lovely ways. Fine . . . but I say, let's at least get something out of it. Let's at least learn something from our trip to the dark side.

How, you ask?

THE "ME/NOT ME" GAME (PARENTING EDITION)

The me/not me game is a simple idea but not easy to incorporate, and (much like the first task I gave you) frankly feels a little weird in the beginning. Like everything related to health and happiness, it is about making the game a practice. (And later, when I get into the putting-this-all-into-practice section, you'll learn all about my Small Steps approach to sustainable change—tools you'll need to make the me/not me game a regular fixture in your life.)

Remember the first task you completed some pages back? The parent you actually are? The values the *real* you holds? That's the "me" of the me/not me game. Got it? And . . . you know the person who just got home from work all stressed out about some totally—in the grand scheme of things—unimportant thing that happened at work, and therefore snapped at his/her child for no good reason? That's the "not me" of the me/not me game.

Another way to put it: The me = the person you feel good about, that you want to give a "Good job" pat on the back to. The not me = the person whose actions land you in a pool of regret and shame, wearing a Speedo. (Though not for long, if you stick with me. I'm talking about the regret and shame. Not the Speedo.)

Here's how you play the game . . . Steal a few moments throughout the day to take an inventory of the times when you were yourself and when you were not yourself. A great time to do this is just before bed. You're (in theory) calm, relaxed, quiet, and can say, "Okay, this morning, when Clarence offered to give me a hand, and I snapped at him because I was tired and irritable? That wasn't me. The me would've accepted his help and thanked him." Then . . . "Later, when I went to grab one of the doughnuts that Brenda had brought to the office but didn't because I re-alized I really didn't want it and would regret it if I ate it? That was me."

What's missing from the "me/not me" scenario? "I'm a crappy person" (self-abuse), "I failed" (self-abuse), or, even worse, "That's just who I am" (too exhausted to self-abuse).

What's *not* missing from the "me/not me" scenario: learning what *you* would've done in the same situation. This creates a real chance of a different outcome next time around. Plus, you might end up apologizing to poor old Clarence, who, incidentally, cried himself to sleep last night. Nice going. He was only trying to help.

Sound weird? Consider this truth: Much of what we've come to think of as "who we are" is made up of behaviors that were instilled in us before we made actual choices about ourselves. During the earliest years of our lives, we soak up both what we're told about who we are and the behaviors our own parents model for us. Ever said to yourself, "Holy crap, I sound exactly like my parents"? That. We're shaped before we do any of our own shaping or have any say in the matter.

But eventually, ideally, we begin to shape our own lives, and as we learn more about who we really are, the more shaping gets done. At the same time, who we really are often lies way beneath and even in conflict with what we were told early on about ourselves. In a sense, we are living lives that aren't ours. But we can break free and, at the very least, begin a transition to living life on our terms.

But we have to set our terms.

Call me an idealist (please), but I believe that deep down, each of us really does know who we are. We just may not be living as that person as much as we'd like to, especially when jobs/family/responsibilities/ stress come flooding in. We don't have the time to bring that person out of hiding. Or so we think.

Which is why . . . in the first task, if with one hand you wrote, "I set a good healthy-eating example for my child" while holding a Twinkie in the other, then perhaps the way you've been eating isn't lining up with who you really are. (By the way, my laptop autocorrected *twinkie* to ensure that the first letter was capitalized. Respect.) But keep in mind this possibility: the Twinkie might be you—a one-off you aren't sweating because it's not your MOTT. Plus, Junior may not be watching.

Becoming a better parent isn't about becoming a different person. It's doing what it takes to do less of the stuff that isn't actually you.

The me/not me game is a way to take a good look at your life critically, but without criticism. Yes, that makes sense, so *shhh*.

Chances are we'll continue to "mis"-behave. (Kind of makes you think twice about that term, now, doesn't it?) But if we can see those times as merely doing something that's really not us, it presupposes that we know who we really are. Then we have a fighting chance to avoid that behavior in the future.

Or, better yet, change the circumstances that might have led to the "mis"-behavior in the first place . . .

Here is how I used the game in my own life, and what I learned . . .

When I walk in the door at the end of the day, I can be distracted and irritable. The last two things I want to be when I come home to my family. And what a great thing to know. Why? Because the fact that I don't want to be those things means being distracted and irritable doesn't line up with *me*. They're not who I am. When I behave that way, I'm not being myself. What remains is to identify the circumstances that trigger those behaviors. In other words, setting the actual behaviors aside, what is at play during the time leading up to my jaunt through the door that sets me off?

I can't tell you how important this is for parents. Actually, I can. Supremely important. All the parenting tools and techniques lining the bookshelves out there are predicated on you being able to implement them. If you don't know who YOU are, then you're looking at an extremely high probability of long-term failure.

The game takes the focus immediately off the behavior and onto a solution.

But back to me/not me and my little irritability problem.

Here is what came up in my effort to identify the circumstances around which I can become irritable: 1) I'm tired, 2) I'm not leaving my work at work, 3) I'm not being productive enough at work, 4) I'm not stealing enough time for myself to reground, reconnect, recover, 5) I've not eaten well (Yes—eat crappy, feel crappy. Feel crappy, be more susceptible to stress. Sorry, but it's true.), 6) I'm pushing myself too hard—during exercise or staying up too late editing a video because I just *have* to get it done . . .

Here's the through line . . . 1–6 have nothing to do with my wife and children and everything to do with my state of mind when I walk through the door. So, I've begun to make little changes to my day, to the life I live, before I walk in the door.

Here are some solutions I'm implementing: 1) Get to sleep earlier, and watch fewer episodes of *The West Wing*, which, incidentally, transports me into a daydream of a world that will never exist, 2) run slower—literally, 3) spend less time on social media, 4) no news watching/listening/website checking.

Take notice. By understanding that being irritable and distracted is not me, I am able to avoid wasting time and energy beating myself up. Then, with that saved time and energy, and the not-feeling-crappy, I'm able to get a good look at what's really going on. Once I notice that, I can take control of the situation by coming up with a course of action. My life/family/children: 1, guilt/shame/criticism: 0. Happier guy, happier father.

Know this: In playing the game, you might come to the realization that your marriage isn't in the best shape and your children aren't super well behaved. Both of these are very real triggers of irritability. But I think that's a darn good thing to know, too. Why? Because, like all the other triggers I listed, you can take steps to improve these. Upping the ante on your family's nutrition, sleep, quality time together, and possibly going to marriage counseling, therapy, or more. All powerful steps you can take once you know. Once you know what you want to get done. To what? To. Make. Your. Family. Happier and healthier.

If you're wondering, "Okay, but how? What are the steps? What food should we be eating?" be patient. We're not there yet. Still setting the stage, but it's a-coming. Stand by for part two of this book. For now, you're just a philosopher sitting on a mountaintop, contemplating the nature of your job as a parent. Nice, calm, deep breaths. But make it quick. That laundry ain't gonna do itself.

LET'S TAKE A MOMENT

Ever seen a video of a lion chasing a zebra? Count out ten seconds in your head. Chances are that chase didn't last much longer than that.

Okay, well, I think I've made my point.

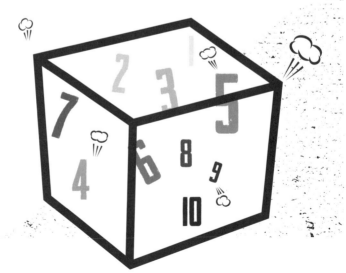

LET'S TAKE ANOTHER MOMENT

Wait—turns out I've got more to say about that now-classic zebra anecdote . . .

When the zebra is chased, it is under stress. The zebra's body takes over in order to survive. It spends zero time weighing options. (Hmmm, should I turn right or left?) It goes on autopilot to escape or fight. But . . . after that ten seconds, the stress is over. Done. For one of two reasons: 1) It's dead (big assumption here, I know, but I'm assuming death is comparatively stress-free—work with me here, will ya?), or 2) it escaped.

Let's focus on option 2 to avoid this book taking a morbid turn.

So, the zebra escapes and rejoins its herd. And the lion doesn't take out a personal vendetta against that particular zebra. It doesn't point at it and exclaim, "I'm coming back just for you, and only you, pal!" By managing to escape, the zebra has bought itself some time. Time to recover.

But enough about the zebra.

Humans have a stress response, too. When we *perceive* stress, our bodies also take over to survive. Some very cool things happen as part of our stress response: increased heart rate, increased blood pressure, stored energy released into the blood, slowed digestion, weakened immune system, mitigated bodily repair, dilated pupils. This is all automatic, instantaneous, and for one purpose: to stay alive until the stress is over. We see the figurative lion and our body effectively shuttles "us" out of the room so it can do its business uninterrupted. "Just read your *People* magazine and keep quiet so I can, you know, keep us alive," it says. Literally.

By the way, notice in the previous paragraph that I put *perceive* in italics? That's because most stress response is triggered by something we believe is stressful. If we see the lion, we'll likely go into stress mode because of what we know about lions. But what if that lion turns out to be Aslan? I mean, that would be the opposite of a stressful situation.

It's how *we* see it. How *we* interpret what's in front of us.

When we think something in the world is harmful or negative, we send a little note to our body that says, "Hey, body, this thing is stressful." Which means . . . something that is stressful to you may not be stressful to me, and vice versa. For example, you and I can be sitting in the same traffic, but one of us isn't in a hurry, slept great the night before, and is listening to our favorite CD, while the other is late for a meeting, tired, and driving a 1985 Chevy Nova with no CD player. Same traffic, two different experiences. You'll read why this is super relevant in a bit.

In the meantime, back to human stress . . .

Every single person I've either worked with or taught reports that they're under significant stress. Yet 99.9 percent of them also report that the stress isn't life threatening in any way—it's job stress, financial stress, relationship stress, commuting stress, etc. Though there was one guy who said he had had life-threatening stress once in 1976. So . . . there was that. But let's just agree most people aren't chased by lions.

So, here we are in such a modern, technologically advanced society that we don't even have to get off our comfy chairs to change a channel, much less forage for our own food and find shelter. And yet we're under stress like nobody's business.

So, what gives?

What gives is that because we've sent the message (picked up by our hypothalamus, pituitary, and adrenals) that there is something stressful afoot, our bodies kick in the same effects as if we were being chased by a lion. Remember the effects? Weakened immune system, weakened digestion, increased blood pressure, increased heart rate, etc., etc.

That's all as it should be. Like the zebra's body, our bodies do an excellent job of keeping us alive during times of stress.

But here's where we and the zebra part ways (and it ain't the stripes).

The zebra has momentary, irregular one-off periods of stress and then—assuming survival—plenty of time to recover. Most humans don't get that time. After our stressful commute comes our stressful job, comes bills to pay, comes being on hold with our cell phone company, comes too much caffeine, comes junk food, comes a sick child or pet, comes too little or poor-quality sleep, comes a breakneck workout at the gym, comes a few beers or worse. We're pummeled by the stress of the modern world and don't have nearly enough time to fully recover before we're hit again. Repeated spikes of stress with not nearly enough nonstress time in between.

Ladies and gentlemen, meet chronic stress.

Chronic stress is repeated spikes of stress with insufficient recovery time. And therefore, this means chronically high blood pressure, chronically weakened immune system, chronic digestive issues, etc. Add to that a gathering of fat around the midsection under chronic stress, and you're seeing the emergence of the modern human.

Fear not—I have a great idea that will solve all our issues resulting from chronic stress. For every fifty-one weeks of stress, we take a one-week vacation. Of course, the one week includes at least two travel days, which are never a walk in the park. With possible jet lag, maybe one more day to acclimate before we start relaxing. That leaves four to five days. That should definitely be sufficient recovery time to offset the fifty-one weeks of modern living.

To be fair, those fifty-one weeks do include the weekends. Two wonderful and full days to recharge, spend some relaxing time with our families, and sleep. Thank goodness for weekends!

Wait . . .

There are errands, soccer games, laundry, chores, bills. We do get to sleep in, however. Wait, not if we have young children or dogs (or a horse).

And so . . .

I believe these two things: 1) To be better parents, we need to figure out how to build more recovery time into our lives, and 2) achieving this will come down to moments.

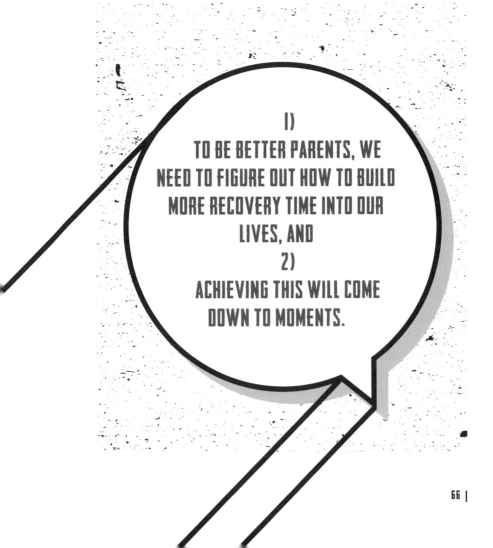

MOMENTS

A few relaxing hours on weekends are fantastic, but not enough. A one-week vacation is fantastic (or so I've heard), but not enough.

Hear this: Your success as a parent hinges on your ability to steal moments of recovery throughout your day. Every day. No more looking to the weekend or to the vacation. We simply can't match our stress to recovery in equal parts. We can't assume an hour of recovery for every hour of stress. But we can learn to be on the lookout for moments. We can create a practice whereby we notice moments we can take for ourselves in places we didn't notice before.

Why "steal"? Because these moments will not be handed to you. Unless . . . I find it interesting that smokers are granted regular and periodic breaks to step outside for a cigarette. Perhaps nonsmokers should pretend they smoke so they, too, can get these breaks throughout the day. Something to think about. Just grab that cigarette-pack-look-alike gum and tell your boss you've got a new nicotine addiction. The only other option would be to tell your boss you're stepping outside for a few minutes to breathe fresh air, reground, and remind yourself of who you are. Yeah, that's not gonna happen.

This is a different way to approach your life.

It's no longer seeing work as work and days off as days off. It's finding time in the middle of anything and everything you're doing.

Here are just a few places you could steal a moment or two of recovery:

- Just before you turn on the news on your morning commute
- On your walk from the car to the office, just before the madness sets in
- In the bathroom (sorry, but a moment of peace is a moment of peace)

- Just before diving into your lunch—or any other meal, for that matter
- While you're waiting for your morning coffee to finish brewing or, if you don't know what's good, your morning tea to finish steeping
- While brushing your teeth
- During a commercial break
- On a run, walk, or mini-trampoline . . . music and podcasts are fun while exercising, but shutting off the iPhone for thirty seconds of deep breathing ain't gonna break the bank.

The fact is that as much as we feel like we "don't have a free moment," we actually do. A bunch of them. When we say "free moment," we're thinking too big. If we actually mean a moment, we've got hundreds in a day.

But here's the argument against taking moments.

They aren't significant-enough chunks of time to make a difference. And I couldn't *dis*agree more.

You might think that meditation is forty-five minutes on a pillow staring at a frickin' candle. I think meditation is being in the moment, present, here. No matter how long you do it. Such that a few intentional deep breaths bring you out of the clusterf&*k of hypothetical conversations, worries, replayed arguments, loud (but wonderful, of course) children, and Muzak versions of "Light my Fire" that are swirling around in your head and into the now.

Okay, so I went hippie there for a spell.

Point is, if you can come into your life during the few minutes you're waiting in line for your coffee, that's a few minutes less of mind chatter.

And even better . . .

If you can steal a few moments in your car, just before you get out and go into the house, it may be just enough to bring you back to you. The real you. You know, the one who walks into the house and *isn't* a ball of stress from the day at work. The one who *isn't* irritated and snappish.

See?

And that was absolutely not a reference to me. I was talking about a friend.

As awesome as cell phones and iPads are, the downside is that they allow us to move through our lives without having to think. To really think. To contemplate, consider, assess. To ask ourselves whether we're actually happy. It's too easy to grab our phone and watch a video or read the news. It's too easy to call a friend, watch a show, or turn on music in the car. But none of those things is essential. They're fun, and we definitely need distractions, to be sure. But *Game of Thrones* is not essential. And I'm not even advising you to stop doing any of those things. For now, only to entertain (pun intended) the idea of grabbing little amounts of time away from those activities—delaying the start of *Game of Thrones* by two minutes—for you.

Worst-case scenario? You do it and it makes no difference. Fine. Curse me and burn this book.

But before you do . . .

Two points: 1) Building a practice of treating yourself better is long term. Unlike quick-fix programs, the results of my approach come with time. 2) You still get to watch *Game of Thrones*.

We all have times when we hit the wall. We've had it, we want it to change, and we want it now. Game on. I'm sick of feeling this way or being overweight, or having the house look like a war zone. We want the solution that will fix things as quickly as possible.

Then, we give up a ton in our efforts to solve these problems. If we're overweight, it means changing what we eat overnight, missing social engagements (or at least making them a lot less fun), making food our overwhelmingly main concern, pissing off the family, and making ourselves miserable. Forget about moments. We go big. Too big. We make sweeping changes. We push, and we push hard.

Is it any wonder this doesn't last? It's exhausting.

AS FAST AS POSSIBLE

Instead, look for moments. You don't abruptly give up *Game of Thrones* because you have to meditate for two hours per day. You take it easy on yourself, and in time your life does improve. And when it does, it's real and long lasting. Living in moments gets you to the change you want. Living in moments keeps you in the change you want. Living in moments doesn't create dysfunction and upset for your family.

But approaching change this way doesn't feel fast enough. The weight doesn't come off as fast as it does with the diet/pill regimen your coworker is doing. The house doesn't get organized fast enough.

Apples and oranges.

Approaching your life and family this way creates actual/lasting change, connecting you to the process in a way that diets or quick fixes never do. Your focus stops being entirely on the finish line. You are aware of your own stress during the process—keeping it at a minimum so you don't cause damage on your way to the finish line. This makes for change that truly does happen as fast as possible.

You get where you want to go nice and easy. And . . . as you do, you walk in the door feeling less irritable. Boom.

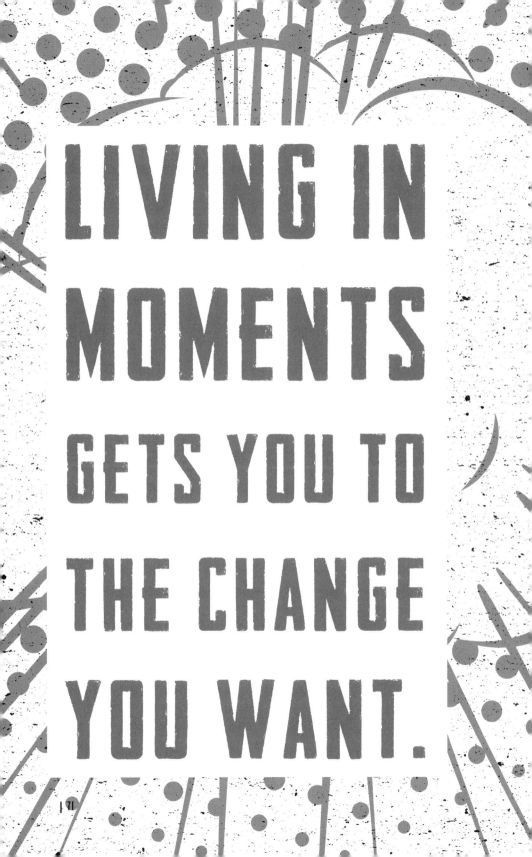

LIVING IN MOMENTS GETS YOU TO THE CHANGE YOU WANT.

PROBLEMS VS. SOLUTIONS

Is junk food your "problem"? Is beer your "problem"? Is TV your "problem"? Have you ever said, "My problem is cheese"?

What if I told you that beer, junk food, TV, and cheese are solutions, not problems. Try seeing these things as what they actually are.

We've tasked ourselves with trying to raise healthy and happy families while getting nailed daily by the nutty nut nut stress of the world. Cracking a beer at the end of the day *is* a solution to that stress. TV, too. Junk food, too. What's better at the end of a crappy day than a cheese pizza? These things really do give us a break. They give us something to look forward to. The question is only whether they're the best solutions, or even kind-of-okay solutions. But let's be clear about the role they play in our lives.

Seeing our so-called problems as solutions means we can assess how effective they are in alleviating our overall stress. Smoking weed surely gives us a break from stress, but is it a good long-term solution?

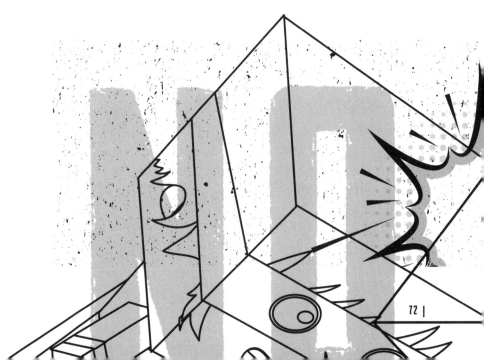

Does it actually alleviate stress for real, or just put it on the back burner for a few hours? Does it make us healthy and happy long term? Does it help us live fulfilling and happy lives?

By recognizing what the solutions are in your life, you may not be so quick to get rid of them all at once. It is fantastic to make the choice to feed yourself and your family better, but remove all the "solution" food tonight, and you'll be facing a mutiny.

You'll be removing that fun before you replace it with new fun.

Instead, you might ease your way in by introducing new, healthier foods little by little. Healthier foods move in slowly, junk foods move out slowly. Time. Change that isn't abrupt, crazy-making, stressful. It is fluid, under-the-radar, subtle. You buy yourself some time to settle on other and better solutions. Your family's health improves along the way, and the stress of the transition to healthier eating is minimized. Win-win.

I never want to take cheese pizza away from your family. Just to show them a way to not need it so much.

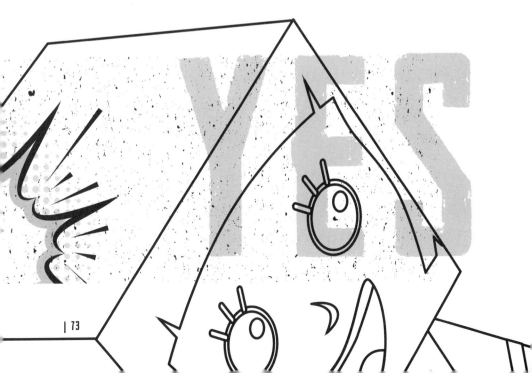

DON'T RECYCLE

Spoiler alert. This is nearly the last part of the first half of my second book. That sentence confused you, and your guard is now down. Too much math, I get it. But now I can get into your head. These aren't the droids you're looking for.

We may not want to admit it, but we channel our parents from time to time. This can be a bad or good experience (depending on how well we think our parents did as parents), but behaviors, habits, words, sayings, songs, even movements can make us go, "Holy crap, I'm frickin' channeling my mom right now."

In the big scheme of things, not a problem, unless it takes the form of fraternity hazing.

Wait, what?

Did I just go off the rails? No, I'm squarely on the rails. Hear me out.

Fraternity brothers traditionally haze pledges for, really, one reason: because they themselves got hazed. It's how it's always been. It's an unquestioned reality. You join up, you know it's coming. You know if you get through it, the tides will change in your favor. Very soon, you will be the hazer, not the hazee. (Yes, it's a word.)

A close friend of mine is a doctor. Her experience during residency? Exhaustion, fatigue, stress. Way overworked and way underpaid. During this period, we invited her over for dinner. She was running late, so we called. She had fallen asleep, but she assured us she was on her way. Never showed, because she fell back to sleep immediately after hanging up.

Why do MDs get put through the ringer during residency when the fatigue is not conducive to learning or performance? It's how it's always been.

Humans are super good at continuing the cycle of behaviors. It's much easier to do than to break the cycle.

Remember, we're wired for easy.

When it comes to our children, however, continuing the cycle of parenting may not be the best thing, and, in fact, may be the exact opposite of the best thing. Unquestioningly, behaving like our parents is really a roll of the dice. If they were good parents, you'll pass that on. If not, you'll pass that on, too.

It's human nature, right? *Ritual de lo habitual.* We continue a habit and sometimes don't even know where it started. It happened to us, and we pay it forward.

One hitch.

I don't think it's human nature. "Human nature" implies a reality we can't change. It says it is how we're wired, so don't question it, and certainly don't waste your time trying to change it.

But we can change our habits. We can break the cycle by not automatically passing our behaviors on to our children. It takes work, focus, struggle, attention. The payoff is huge—you become the parent you're meant to be.

Perhaps human nature is our ability to adapt, to change, to make choices. To think. To create. Time to raise the bar.

Are you ready for it? Before saying yes, know that you might need to decrease the time you spend on CNN or Fox News, Facebook, and Twitter by a few minutes. I know you can do it.

"Example is not the main thing in influencing others. It is the only thing."

— ALBERT SCHWEITZER

HEADLINE NEWS: SCHWEITZER NAILS IT

I love *and* hate Schweitzer's quote.

I love it because it's frickin' true.

I hate it because it's frickin' true.

Everything you've read so far, and what follows, comes down to this truth. To this pill that is tough to swallow.

That when we get down to it, to the foundation of everything we know about ourselves and our children—beneath the veil, behind the curtain—it comes down to this:

Your children are shaped more by the example you set than by any parenting technique you'll ever know.

I began this book with the section title "It's All About You." Up to this point, I've written almost entirely about you, your happiness, your goals, your dreams. The parent YOU truly are.

We, as parents, can make it all about our kids, and if we do, we will pursue all the parenting and diet books in the world. With the best of intentions. For our kids. We want to enable and empower our children to succeed in this nutty nut nut world, and if we can just find the magic bullet of communication, teaching method, disciplinary system, we are absolutely sure we can lock this down.

And all the while, we put our own happiness on the back burner. Our own health on the back burner.

And our children watch.

They see not only a parent who isn't super happy and super healthy but also a parent who isn't putting a priority on either. A parent who, regardless of what he or she says, doesn't seem to think health and happiness are really all that important.

Dang.

DO AS I SAY, NOT AS I DO

Really?

Whoever came up with that saying was really striving for excellence. Not.

We want happy and healthy children. We want them to know how to take care of themselves. We want them to be strong and know that they'll be able to kick ass.

Do you really think they're going to learn that from the book *we* read and used to teach them?

This idea—that the example we set is first and foremost (well, Albert says, the "only," and he won a Nobel Prize) in how we influence our children—is so simple. We get it. Not hard to understand conceptually.

But when push comes to shove, it is a tough pill to swallow because the burden of change weighs heavy on our shoulders. In an odd way, it is easier to instruct, to project, to deflect. To look outward to our children.

"It doesn't matter that I am overweight, as long as I teach my child about healthy eating," except it totally does matter.

"It doesn't matter that I hate my job and come home every night in a bad mood, as long as I provide them the resources—education, for instance—to enable them to live a happy life," except it totally does matter.

"It doesn't matter that I don't exercise, am tired, and watch a ton of television, as long as I tell my kid to go outside and play," except it totally does matter.

Telling your child to go to college may get them to college. Telling your child to eat a salad may get them to eat a salad. But if health and happiness are your umbrella goals, it may be time to "do as I say *and* as I do."

Boom.

THE SUBTLE SINK-IN

There's a subtlety to my approach to healthy families. Strapping a Mozart band around your pregnant belly isn't subtle. I'm not saying don't go ahead and strap away, by the way. I'm just saying it is not subtle.

Becoming a better example for your child doesn't make a huge difference overnight.

Understand that the example you set begins with the decision to be a better example. If you want to be a better example of health, you eat better and start exercising. Your child sees that and learns from it long before your stomach flattens out. You're parenting well by virtue of what you're *becoming*.

What do or will your children see when they look at you? Do they see the real you? Something close to that parent you described in the first task I gave you (see page 38), or one that is at least trying to get there?

Children live many years with us. Years. Years of seeing how we live, what we eat, how we communicate, how happy or unhappy we are, if we love or hate the work we do. On isolated days, we might be happy, we might eat a healthy meal, but over years? Subtle.

Our children don't consciously decide that they're going to be influenced by the example we set. It's under the radar. It's pretty much unintentional. It happens with little or no effort at all. We live, they soak it up. How we live is up to us, but that our children internalize our lives is already happening and out of our control.

Hypothetical: You tell your child that you're tired of being unhealthy and are going to make an effort to take better care of yourself. Then you actually do make the effort. It's not much at first, but it's real and quantifiable. You toss your potato chips in the trash. You tell your child you're going for a walk outside. A five-minute walk. Your child sees this.

Here's what your child sees:

- Strength
- Integrity
- Independence
- Self-confidence
- Self-esteem
- Self-respect
- Happiness
- Action

And they're seeing it on day one. And days two to five thousand. It's sinking in, and it's subtle. Sure, eventually they'll see a flat stomach, but what they see before that time is way more valuable. Way more.

Here's the kicker. It actually doesn't matter if you never get the flat stomach. The end result makes little difference. Just shooting for personal happiness and health sends your child the message that happiness and health are possibilities. If they weren't, why would you even try?

Leap of faith here, but give this a shot and your life will change on day one. You'll immediately be healthier and happier in mind. Your body will follow. You will experience true change. It's subtle, yes, but you'll take notice.

What does your child see right now? Me, or not me?

EALIT

TYRE

EALIT

TYRE

REALITY
LITY R
REALI
LITY R

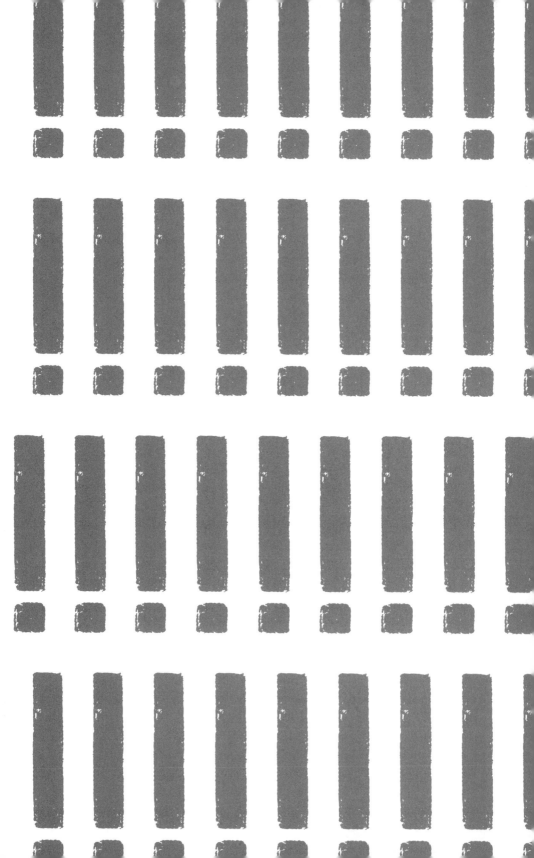

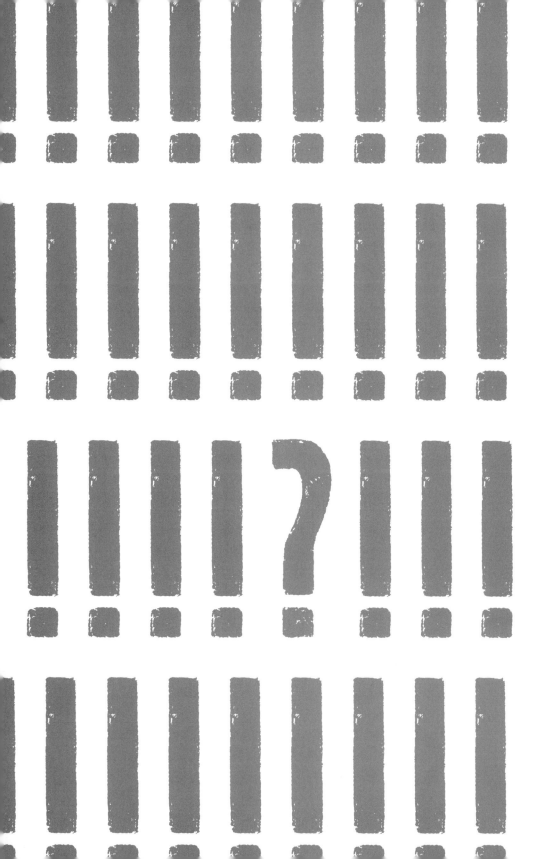

WELCOME TO REALITY

A strong foundation of knowledge in place. A clear idea of what your ideal family dynamic looks like. A clear idea of your ideal parenting approach. Now it is time to act. Now it is time to move your life and your family closer to your ideal.

What follows in these pages are tools that empower you to make changes. Real and long-lasting changes. Not spikes of change that last only a short time before everything returns to how it used to be.

But first . . . a few things to consider that will help you get the changes going, especially in the beginning.

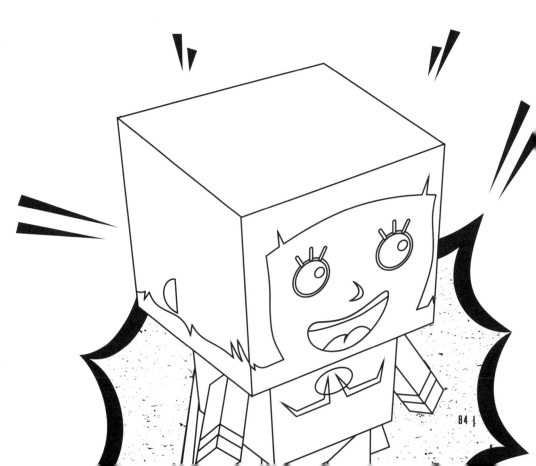

THE STRUGGLE OF THE MUGGLE

Hopefully, in the Philosophy section, you understood that transition-
ing your family to greater health and happiness is a process. It takes
work. It takes attention. There is struggle.

I have coached many people in my Small Steps approach, and not
once have I ever tried to convince someone that change comes easy.
It doesn't. Diets are easy. Quick fixes are easy. To be sure, they do take
work, but most have an end date such that no matter how difficult a
plan is to execute, we know the difficulty won't last for very long. And
when the last day of the diet arrives, chances are your old life will come
flooding back in, and any progress made will be undone.

Not so with real change. It is ongoing, and there is a very real
struggle associated with it. No infomercial here. Just reality.

My goal isn't to sell you on an effortless transition to a healthy
family. My goal is to empower you to embrace the struggle more fully
and to understand this super-important point:

It is the struggle itself that leads to happiness.

Soon, I will get into the nitty-gritty of my Small Steps approach, but
. . . spoiler alert:

While my approach doesn't remove the struggle, it minimizes it like
nobody's business.

Incidentally, Hermione nails my Small Steps approach, and she's
Muggle-born. (Did you really think, after seeing this section's header, I
wasn't going to reference Muggles?)

THE TENSION OF "SHOULD"

I've come to loathe the word *should* (and its evil twin, *shouldn't*). I wish it could be removed from the language for good, but in the meantime, I'm working to minimize its usage. Why? Because it's an unnecessary pressure. It implies that anything you *should* be doing is something you can't actually be doing right now. It implies a self-criticism and a negativity we'd all be better off without.

If you think there is something you *should* be doing, take away the "should" and start doing it. That is, if you *want* to start doing it. Chuck the "should" so you can ask yourself whether you want to. Better yet, ask whether the parent in your first task is already doing it. Remember the first-task parent? Notice that he/she isn't bogged down with "should"s.

This goes for all the information you're going to get in this section. The food, the movement, the small steps. Everything. No "should"s allowed. Take on what you want to take on. Choose it or don't. If you hear yourself saying, "I really should do what he's suggesting," ask yourself why. Why should you? Because you think I'm saying you should?

Instead, try, "That sounds cool—I'd like to do it." Or, "Nah, that isn't for me."

To illustrate, what follows is a brilliant one-act play that also provides a little glimpse into my Small Steps approach . . .

Someone: I *should* eat healthier.

Me: Why?

Someone: Well, because I want to set a better example for my child, and because I want to be at a good weight, have more energy, etc.

Me: Okay, so you *want* to eat healthier.

Someone: Well, yes. Seems like such a massive undertaking, though. I'd have to give up the food I love. Plus, I do the cooking but don't want to force this on my family, so I'd have to make a separate meal for myself on top of what I make for the family.

Me: Who said anything about a massive undertaking?

Someone: Well, isn't it?

Me: Can you include a couple stalks of celery with whatever you eat for dinner tonight?

Someone: Yeah, that's super easy.

Me: Then you'll be eating healthier, starting today.

Someone: Two stalks of celery won't do squat.

Me: This isn't about weight loss yet. Just start with the celery. Get used to putting some healthy food in your body every day. Start *thinking* of yourself as someone who puts healthy food in his/her body every day. This immediately shows your child that you are making an effort to improve your life by taking real action. See? The celery is doing a ton. Later, the celery will turn into a side salad, will turn into a morning smoothie, will turn into whole-grain pasta, will turn into a big frickin' salad for dinner. Later, your weight will come down as your health goes up.

Someone: Dang.

Me: Right? Totally.

And . . . scene.

"Should" is pressure on us that has no business being there. Pressure that keeps us from taking the very action we think we *should* be doing.

COMPARED TO WHAT?

If you choose to incorporate some of the actions/tasks/tools in this book, change will come.

To be successful with any transition, change, or transformation, it is imperative to stay focused on you—or, in this case, you and your family. Too often, we look over to the next guy/gal/family to see how we're measuring up. That is a losing endeavor. Too hard to get the whole picture, anyways. Kind of like thinking you are getting an in-depth look at your friend's life from his Facebook posts. It ain't the whole picture, so don't bother trying. It's time best spent elsewhere.

Instead, and as much as possible, measure your success in isolation. Time spent comparing yourself to others is time spent away from the actual work of improving your life. And, more important, time spent away from feeling good about the improvements you are already making.

The person in the next cubicle, who is on day eighteen of some twenty-one-day frickin' gummy-bear diet, may be a lot slimmer than he/she was eighteen days ago. You, on the other hand, are easing your

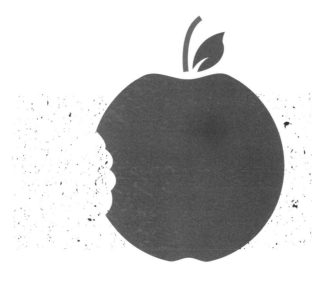

way in with healthier eating. Creating new habits. Keeping your stress low. Understanding the long-term nature of what you're taking on. Incredible. But, dang, that person has lost so much weight! You *should* be losing more weight by now, right?

Apples and oranges.

Your coworker is on a very short train ride. No new habits, no new self-knowledge, burning through their willpower in the meantime, and most likely gaining the weight back.

Compare yourself to that person on his day eighteen? Of course you feel inadequate.

Keep your eye on the ball of what you are actually accomplishing, and you feel like a champion.

So . . . Keeping up with the Joneses ain't the name of the game when you're working for a healthier, happier family.

Unless your last name is Jones.

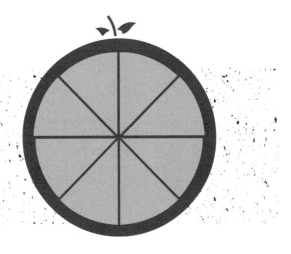

A REFRESHING LOOK AT STRESS

For a time at UCLA, I titled all my philosophy papers "A Refreshing Look at [insert name of philosopher or philosophy]." Didn't seem to do much for my GPA, but it's still inexplicably funny to me.

In the Philosophy section, I addressed stress. Namely, the effects of stress and how we, as parents, need to be on the lookout for moments to decrease our own overall stress.

I am revisiting the subject here for a reason. Because in the following pages, I will be getting deeper into nutrition, meals, healthy eating in general, and I want to make sure you know and remember this crucial fact:

Food is just one of the things that can aid us in our quest to live better and, likewise, just one of the things that can prevent us from living better.

I want to drive this point home because . . .

Time and time again, people conceptually understand the idea that health and happiness are a broad picture, and yet, when they learn about food/nutrition, all of a sudden, too much of their attention goes to food. When it does, it is at the expense of the rest of their lives. I have seen many people spend an inordinate amount of time thinking about food—carrying lists of foods they can and can't eat, and doing everything they can to ensure that there's ne'er a stray-away from their self-imposed rules (or, worse, rules imposed by a guru). No big surprise, but they're not living a vibrant, thriving, happy life. One can only imagine the effect this has on their friends and family.

So . . .

What you'll learn in this book about healthy eating can serve you and your family extremely well but can also throw your family into turmoil. If you want to know why, reread the first section. Dig?

Here's the thing about stress. It can be awesome. A little goes a long way in helping us grow and evolve physically and mentally.

The stress that can pull this off? Adaptive stress.

This is the kind of stress that is *just* enough stress to allow our minds and bodies to play catch-up.

To illustrate:

I've run my entire life but have never been a good, much less a great, runner. Certainly not a super-long-distance runner. Yet, at forty-six years old, I ran my first two trail ultramarathons. (FYI, an ultramarathon is any distance over a 26.2-mile marathon.) In fact, it was only one year before the ultras that I had run my first marathon.

Having no experience whatsoever with a trail ultra, I read up on the subject, then got some help from a coach for a few months. The single greatest thing I learned?

Slow down. To slow down more than I ever had. Ever.

This was easier said than done. Again, I'd run my entire life. Much shorter distances, but I could maintain a fairly decent clip. And yet, time and time again, I came across the same advice. Slow down, almost to an embarrassing pace.

My main goal wasn't to win my first, or any, ultramarathon.

My goal was to finish the damn race and finish strong, so I decided to give it a try.

Here's the "why" of training slow. It minimizes the stress of the run, thus allowing your body to adjust to the distance. Keep your Most-of-the-Time slow (What?!? Yep, MOTT here, too), and you can increase your distance over time without paying for it.

Go out too fast and too hard, and you cause too much stress, forcing your body to do just what it needs to get through that particular run, without the necessary adaptations and adjustments that enable improvements in efficiency and endurance.

As I ran slower, I found myself able to run much longer distances without the soreness and fatigue that had plagued me even during the previous year's marathon training, before I had learned about slowing down. No injuries, no sickness, no fatigue. Training *and* having the energy to spend time with family.

Keep your stress levels low enough, and you change for the better. Keep them high, and you plateau.

Under high stress, you get by. You survive, but you don't thrive.

So, same goes for the family. A high-stress family life is solely about getting through the needs of the day. Getting by. Treading water. Forget about improving your family's health and happiness. You're over-whelmed enough as it is. Literally "over" "whelmed."

I just pretended to know what *whelm* means. Nailed it.

So . . .

Use the information that follows in a way that keeps the stress at the adaptive level. As in not debilitating.

Take on more than you and your family are ready to take on, and you might as well not take it on in the first place . . .

How do you know whether you're taking on too much at once? Unhappy family. Daily dysfunction. Daily arguments. Outright rebellion. That's how you know.

How do you know whether you're taking on the right amount of stress? A spirit of adventure, experimentation, curiosity in your family. Open communication. A "Hey, let's try this" approach. No shoving anything down anyone's throats. Fun.

I'll repeat this point: If you want change, you probably want it super fast. Get 'er done. But this drive can lure you into taking on too much at once. Do this, and there's a good chance your family will burn out. You won't be able to sustain the stress, and eventually it won't be worth it.

Just so you know, my approach will create the changes you want AS FAST AS POSSIBLE. Literally—you are in control of maintaining the quantity and speed of the changes such that long-term success is achievable.

TO SLOW DOWN MORE THAN I EVER HAD.

MIDTERM
TABLE OF
CONTENTS
MIDTERM

Think it's odd to have a table of contents appear for no particular reason? Me, too. Never stopped me before.

This is a breakdown of what follows so you can jump to sections as needed, but the CliffsNotes version is this: I handily convince you of my nutrition approach, my movement approach, my stuff-for-the-mind approach, then jump fully into implementation via my Small Steps approach to habit/behavior change (as applied to children as well, of course). In other words, know, then act.

HEAVY-BOX NUTRITION

Food. We love it.

Wow, what a great slogan—just not sure for what company.

Humans love food so much, we've figured out a way to manipulate it to such an extent that it has become addictive. Think you're a binger, a chronic overeater? Sit down in front of a big, huge bowl of PLAIN lettuce (no dressing/oil/spices), and eat with reckless abandon. Here's what will happen. You WON'T binge. You WON'T overeat. The lettuce is natural, unadulterated, and you and your body understand it. It makes sense. It nourishes, hydrates, satisfies *actual* hunger without, well, lighting your head on fire.

My point is this: Along with our ability to make food taste super good via processing, combining, cooking, spicing, and flavoring came the expectation that our food should *always* taste super good. Frankly, unnaturally good. The lettuce above probably tastes just fine to most people, but compared to Cap'n Crunch (with Crunchberries, since studies have shown berries to be extremely nutritious), it just doesn't cut it. We've raised the taste bar so significantly (and our taste buds came along for the ride) that any idea of eating more simply and naturally literally isn't on the table.

This is the greatest challenge I have in my work. Communicating the truth about healthy eating: It's extremely simple and easy.

Challenge accepted.

I hear people all the time say, "It's really hard to eat healthy," "You have to spend so much more time in the kitchen," etc. Not true. But alas . . .

What follows is my approach to nutrition/healthy eating. The MOTT from the first section comes into play big-time here because I love food, my family loves food. We eat healthy AND enjoy food. We are not silently sitting around a table eating plain lettuce, scowling at each other as we chew incessantly for hours on end, eating our misery.

But . . .

Fact is, we do eat pretty simply most of the time. Not bland, not plain, but simply. Later in this section, there will be awesome recipes to try, but for now . . .

FIRST "FOOD AS CAR FUEL," THEN "FOOD AS BOX"—OR "SID, PLEASE JUST SETTLE ON ONE METAPHOR"

Confused? Just wait—you'll be the opposite of confused in a very short time.

First, the definition of *food*: Anything we eat that our bodies convert to usable energy. (As parents, we know full well the plethora of items our children ingest that their bodies can't convert to usable energy, like the dime my daughter swallowed at age three. Not food.) Energy to do the things we are designed to do. For example, walk/run, fight infections, think, digest, detoxify, and talk. Or as I call it, Tuesday.

We invented the concept of the calorie as a measure of that energy, and it comes in three forms: protein, fat, and carbohydrates. These three are also referred to as the macronutrients. And if something is food for us, it has to have one, two, or all three of these macronutrients in a form we can digest.

In addition to the macronutrients in food, there are micronutrients: vitamins, minerals, antioxidants, and phytochemicals (plant compounds that are essential for the health of our bodies/minds). These are not calories, we don't convert them to energy, but they're extremely important.

So, food: a combination of macro- and micronutrients. Different foods have different combinations of these two types of nutrients. But first, let's talk cars . . .

For a car to drive (i.e., to do what it's designed to do), it for sure needs gas. Won't start up without it. But it also needs motor oil. What does motor oil do? Lubricates the engine. Keeps the parts moving well so that while it's burning the gas for the energy it needs to drive, it's not, well, burning out. Put only gas (no oil) in your Ferrari, and you're headed for a breakdown. Put only oil (no gas) in your Ferrari, and you're headed nowhere, because that gorgeous machine won't start.

In other words, for a car to drive *optimally* and for as long as possible, it needs gas AND motor oil.

Now, back to us.

As I wrote earlier, we, too, need an energy source to do what we do, BUT . . . to do what *we* do optimally, and *for as long as possible*, we need the human version of motor oil. Something that keeps the engine running cleanly and efficiently while it burns calories. Enter the micronutrients: vitamins, minerals, antioxidants, and phytochemicals.

In other words, you can have all the protein, fat, and carbohydrates (i.e., fuel) in the world, but if you don't have sufficient micronutrients (the motor oil), your body (the engine) will suffer.

NOW, LET'S TALK ABOUT GIFTS

'm only using two food analogies total, and this is the last one, so calm down, for crying out loud.

Imagine all foods as gifts. Every food is a box with wrapping paper on it. The wrapping paper represents the energy we get from food. The macronutrients. The protein, fat, carbohydrates. The stuff that makes our machine *run*. In other words, anything that is human food has wrapping paper. That's a constant. No matter what food you're talking about (from butter to butter lettuce), it is wrapped in a pretty wrapping paper.

How about inside the box?

The gift inside the box represents the micronutrients. The vitamins, minerals, antioxidants, phytochemicals. The stuff that makes our machine run *well* . . .

Think about what you do when you're given a gift . . . You unwrap it to find out what's inside. You probably don't sit admiring the wrapping paper for too long. You want the goods. You want that which is of value—what's inside the box.

Same with food. Yes, of course we need energy. It's crucial. We need protein, fat, and carbohydrates. We need it to run. But . . . the value of any food is determined by what comes *with* the energy. The gift inside the box. That's what determines how healthy the food actually is.

In other words—the heavier the box, the healthier the food. Not the wrapping paper, but the gift. If you open the gift and there's nothing inside, you've just been handed the worst Christmas ever. AND, irritable bowel syndrome. Wait, what? Sorry, couldn't resist.

If you open the gift and there's awesomeness inside, you're a happy camper.

In keeping with the food as gift-box metaphor, here are the basics, from light or empty boxes to heavy boxes:

In the light-/empty-box corner: processed plants like *added* sugar, oil, white/refined flour, white/refined rice, soy protein isolate. Basically, plants that *used* to be part of a whole, until we got busy extracting, messing with, isolating, inventing. For example, soy protein isolate (found in some fake meats and cheeses and protein powders and bars) *used* to be in a soybean. The soybean HAD protein, fat, carbohydrates, vitamins, minerals, antioxidants, phytochemicals, and more. Soy protein isolate? Almost entirely protein, with a mere fraction of what existed in the whole bean. Processed. Refined. Isolated.

Olive oil *used* to be in an olive. White rice *used* to be brown rice. White flour *used* to be whole wheat. Get it? WE did this. Humans did it. We didn't stumble on an olive oil plant, a white-sugar tree, or a soy-protein-isolate shrub. We take plants that are more natural and make them less natural. Then we make stuff like Twinkies, protein powder, Wonder Bread, and containers of super-hot oil in which we deep-fry *whatever we can.*

A heavier box? Animal foods like dairy, eggs, flesh (fish, turkey, chicken, beef, etc.). As with repurposing plants, humans have also done a bang-up job essentially creating animals that bear little resemblance to anything natural or wild. Feeding corn to a cow is, well, nutty nut nut. So, in moving up the light-box-to-heavy-box spectrum, the more natural the animal, the heavier-box the flesh or breast milk of that animal. In other words, the healthier the animal eats (and, like humans, the less chronically stressed the animal is), the healthier the animal. It ain't brain surgery. The beef you buy at the market isn't in the same ballpark as a wild antelope, much like the bag of sugar isn't in the same ballpark as an orange.

Moving on to heavier pastures.

Next up? Nuts/seeds. Cashews, almonds, hemp, sunflower seeds, walnuts, pumpkin seeds, etc. Heavier boxes than animal foods and refined/processed plants, nuts and seeds have even more of the micronutrients in the calories they deliver. More motor oil with the gas.

and . . . just as important, fiber appears for the first time. Nuts and seeds, along with macro- and micronutrients, have fiber (technically, fibers). Fiber is, for me, so essential that I'm *this* close (picture me holding my thumb and index finger dangerously close) to simply saying that if the food you eat has fiber in it, it's awesome.

Why? Because in addition to what most people understand about fiber—that it helps keep the digestive tract clean and regulates absorption of nutrients into the body (fiber plays an absolutely essential and additional role in the body)—it feeds the good bacteria in our gut. Huge. Big-time. *Importante.* The good bacteria in our gut that aids our sleep, our immune system/inflammatory response, and even our mood. (Remember the first section of the book? Happier parents, happier family. Help us, O bacterial comrades!)

From nuts and seeds, we go even heavier, to whole grains and beans. In this area appear *whole* versions of wheat, barley, rye, kamut, spelt, etc., plus grain-like foods (grain "like" because they're actually seeds) such as quinoa, brown rice, buckwheat, amaranth, wild rice, millet. Also in this arena are beans of all types, like kidney, pinto, adzuki, lentil, black, red, and a whole host of others.

Finishing up in the heaviest-box corner are fruits and vegetables . . .

Short recap:

Lightest-box foods are nutty nut nut, manipulated, unnatural, technology-created foods. Heaviest-box foods are less manipulated, more natural, not nutty nut nut (except for the nuts).

Wow, SO complicated! (Sense the sarcasm?)

Is this a fairly general list? Yes. Could I go way more into detail, listing every vitamin and mineral in every single type of food on the earth? Yes. In fact, see the Resources section if you want to go deeper.

Why don't I?

Because this book is intended to help you and your family frickin' thrive.

The heavier-box the foods the family eats most of the time, the better off those bodies you are all walking around in. Let's not overcomplicate this, okay? Let's not focus just on calories, because every food's got 'em. Instead, let's focus on the whole enchilada.

I'VE GOT TO CONCENTRATE ... CONCENTRATE ... CONCENTRATE ...

A nyone around my age will know that's a reference to the film *Airplane*. I must be getting old, because I find myself having to explain my references more and more these days: "Wait, you've never heard of the Pixies?!?"

Let me try again:

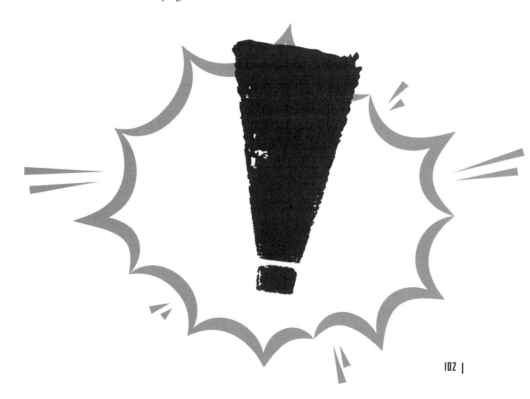

A REFRESHING LOOK AT CALORIC CONCENTRATION

ang. Still doesn't help.

Caloric concentration is one of my most important areas of teaching for anyone interested in healthy eating. The good news is that the light-box-to-heavy-box spectrum helps make sense of it ever so perfectly.

So, what is caloric concentration?

While our focus needs to be more on the gift inside the box and less on the wrapping paper, fact is, our bodies do run off the wrapping paper (cuz it's the gas). What this means is that the health of anyone's diet is determined by the proportion of heavy-box to light-/empty-box calories. Unfortunately, most people look at food incorrectly. They assess food by what it looks like on the plate, how much size it takes up.

Incidentally, what comes next will make portion control look as crazy as it actually is.

Confused? Here comes the clarity . . .

Your body doesn't care about the portion size or shape of what you eat. It just needs fuel to do its job, and it likes it best when it gets just the right amount (and ideally with the healthy stuff, too)—not too much, and not too little. The Goldilocks of caloric intake.

Looking at food through the lens of caloric concentration makes its size and shape irrelevant. Here's why: Compare 120 calories of olive oil (one tablespoon) to 120 calories of lettuce (about two and a half heads of lettuce). Same calories, but couldn't look more different on a plate. So, if you have even 50 calories of lettuce on your plate (about a head of lettuce—substantially more than most have in a salad) and drizzle a couple of tablespoons of olive oil on it (picture a couple of tablespoons—it could fit in the palm of your hand), things aren't what they seem. While the food *looks* like a big plate of lettuce and a tiny bit of olive oil, calorically, it is the opposite: a tiny bit of lettuce with a ton of olive oil on it. Again, calorically.

Get it? Only 50 calories of lettuce, and 240 calories of olive oil. Way more light-box than heavy-box.

Healthy eating ain't about what the food looks like, but about where most of the calories you eat come from.

Kind of twists your noodle a little, no?

Fine, as long as your noodle is whole grain.

Ever heard someone say they eat a lot of fruit because they have half a banana and a handful of blueberries on their oatmeal? Calorically, they're not eating much fruit (about 60 calories), especially in proportion to an average adult's daily caloric intake (2,000 calories). On the other hand, the shake I drink that I make with ten bananas, two cups of frozen berries, and water? That's about 1,100–1,200 calories of fruit. That is a lot of fruit.

If you're still thinking, man, that's a lot of sugar. It is. Awesome sugar. Comes with the stuff that makes my body run well.

It might surprise you that a Big Mac, a six-piece order of Chicken McNuggets, large fries, large coke (or as I called it in high school, "the usual") is almost 1,600 calories, and takes up a heckuva lot less space than my ten bananas. It fits in a nice little bag, and while it may not *look* like a ton of food, trust me, it is. And it, unlike the fruit smoothie, ruins the machine.

Turns out that as you eat heavier-box, you have to eat bigger meals to get the same calories you get from much smaller lighter-box meals. Because a plate with half fried chicken and half green beans is calorically a big ol' fried-chicken meal with a teensy bit of green beans, you'd need to add a huge quantity of green beans to even things up, and would need a second plate to do it.

What does all this mean? It means that eating healthier means understanding that you'll have to eat greater portions of heavy-box foods to get the calories you need to do the stuff you want to do. The size of your meals gets bigger, while the caloric content stays the same.

Weird, right?

Good news? You never feel hungry. You eat until you're full. Like every dang wild animal.

Ever seen a wild gorilla portion control? Ever heard one say, "Gosh, I really want more leaves, but I probably shouldn't."

See the next section, but first . . .

A couple common nutritional mistakes:

1. People move to a predominantly heavy-box diet (lots of fruits and vegetables, with some whole grains, beans, and a bit of nuts/seeds), don't eat big enough portions to get the calories they need, then complain that they had *more energy* when they were eating more animal foods and refined plants (oil, white flour, etc.). Know why? Because they *did* have more *energy* when they were eating those calorically concentrated foods—just not more *health*. The solution is simple: Eat bigger portions of the lower-calorie/healthier/fiber-filled foods.

2. People who just can't figure out why they can't lose weight since they're eating "a ton" of fruits and vegetables. It might look to them like they are, but that eight-ounce glass of fruit smoothie for breakfast ain't gonna cut it in the fruit realm, just as the "big" (but not really big) side salad ain't gonna cut it in the vegetable realm. Most likely, more of their calories are still coming from light-box foods, their bodies aren't running well, and the extra weight they are holding onto is their body telling them so. Grate some cheese on that side salad, add a buttermilk ranch dressing, and it's like you've stopped eating a salad altogether.

MEASURING, COUNTING, AND WEIGHING, OH MY!

In spite of how much you now know about heavier boxes, caloric concentration, macronutrients, micronutrients, and caloric quantity versus quality, I beg you to either stop, or don't start, counting calories or controlling portions. Neither is natural, and (luckily) both become more obsolete, the healthier the food you eat. In my house, if we kept portions small, we would rarely get enough calories, since most of our calories come from heavy-box foods. My salads are HUGE. I call them Big Frickin' Salads for a reason. We eat large portions of food, eat 'til we're full, and are happier for it.

On the other hand, you might be saying to yourself, "Sid, that's all fine and good, but I'm going to stick with my McNuggets, pizza, and fries, and furthermore, sir, you can't tell me what to do!"

First, I'm not telling you what to do. I'm not the boss of you, and one more thing: You're not nine, so let's, you know . . . geesh.

Second, if the McNuggets/pizza/fries extravaganza is your bag, have at it. BUT . . . in that case, I highly recommend you DO count your calories and control your portions. Why? Those "tech foods" pack a wallop. Eating until you are full on light-box foods means a ton of un-healthy calories—and an increased chance of sickness if you don't check yourself (long before you wreck yourself, that is). You'd need to restrict and limit the size of your meal, while mine wouldn't even fit on a plate. See the difference?

Added bonus of eating heavier-box foods? You will NEVER feel hungry. You'll eat large quantities of food and feel kick-ass.

THE FIBER OF OUR LIVES: SOME SIMPLE GUIDELINES

Fiber is the fiber of our lives. Not cotton. There. I said it.

I mentioned fibers earlier and the crucial role they play in our health. Hopefully, by now you know I'm not referring to some nutty nut nut fiber-powder-in-a-jar you mix into water and drink. Jiminy Christmas. What is it with our species? We love to extract, isolate, manipulate. Hey, humans! Leave the stuff that comes in food *in* the frickin' food. Stop taking it out and putting it in pills and jars, for crying out loud.

I mention fiber again here by way of throwing down some very simple nutritional guidelines:

1. Focusing on fiber is a very simple way to look at food without getting sucked down the rabbit hole of macro- versus micronutrients, etc. Food with fiber is better for you than food without.

2. The more natural (i.e., less "messed with") the food, the healthier. A raw cashew has fiber in it, just as a roasted/salted cashew has fiber in it. But the raw one is less messed with, so it ranks higher on the health-o-meter. Whole grains are less messed with than refined grains. An orange is less messed with than orange juice. For that matter, fresh-squeezed orange juice is less messed with than orange juice from concentrate.

3. Don't get into absolutes. It's not that orange juice is bad. It's a heck of a lot better than sodas, just not as healthy as the orange. *Not as.* In general, it's all about where a food sits on the light-box-to-heavy-box spectrum.

I'M STILL AFRAID

I'm still afraid of anyone reading this getting militant about food. Feeling the huge urge to memorize every single food known to humans, assess each one's nutritional makeup, make note of where it sits on the heavy-box spectrum, and then expend energy and time memorizing it.

You can go ahead and give that a shot, but it's going to be a huge and time-consuming undertaking. Make sure you have a caretaker for the children: Mommy and Daddy are going to "be away" for a while.

Instead, how about this additional and awesome bonus to eating heavy-box foods most of the time: You barely have to think about food.

I'm a nutritionist, yet I think less about food than most.

Why?

My family eats the foods that make it so I don't have to.

I'M A NUTRITIONIST, YET I THINK LESS ABOUT FOOD THAN MOST.

SUPPLEMENTS, PILLS, AND BOTTLES, OH MY!

A note on supplementation.

My philosophy of supplementing with vitamin/mineral pills is this: Supplement to match the level of unnatural.

Here's what I mean. If you are still the person referenced above who insists on the McNuggets/pizza/fries trifecta, it's probably a good idea for you to take vitamin/mineral supplements. (In addition to the counting calories and controlling portions. Geesh, what a hassle . . . So restrictive!) Why? Cuz you're not getting enough micronutrients from the food you're eating.

Here is what my family does:

- When we are not in the sun, we take vitamin D.
- Because we neither eat food with dirt on it nor eat animals who eat food with dirt on it, we take vitamin B12. (B12, contrary to popular belief, doesn't originate in meat. If it did, where would the cows get it? Exactly . . . It's a dirt thing.)

That's it. No multivitamins, no multiminerals. D and B12.

If we modern humans were more natural, walking around the forest outside, getting sun on our skin, and eating food directly from the ground, we wouldn't need pills. You know, like the way wild animals don't.

THE FEAR FACTOR

Here's actually one good thing bottles and pills do: alleviate fear. With a bottle of calcium capsules, you can read exactly how much you're getting. It's measurable, quantifiable, and much more exacting than sesame seeds. (Good source of calcium, by the way, like most heavy-box foods.)

Couple little, teensy-weensy, totally unimportant points here:

1. The calcium in the capsule is no longer in its natural state. (And has been separated from the other vitamins and minerals with which it was coexisting. So sad!) Sure, you can see how many milligrams from the label, but how do you know how much of that 1,200 mg is actually going to be absorbed and utilized by your body? Ever wonder why people in the United States take in so much calcium but have some of the worst bone health in the world? Health is a bigger picture than any single nutrient: Go broader and eat food with more of the stuff.

2. Mother Nature isn't stupid. While we have the brains and technology to extract and isolate nutrients, we haven't outsmarted her. Nutrients are still best when left in their natural state. Period. Mother Nature: "I already made food for you. Why do you insist on changing it? Don't you have anything better to do? Now, clean your room and go outside and play."

Actually, those points weren't teensy-weensy. They speak to a real issue with parenting and healthy families: fear.

We are afraid that we won't provide the right nutrition for our families. The fear doesn't feel good. So . . .

We are willing to spend money to minimize that fear, but often at the expense of our health and happiness.

Afraid your child is not getting enough protein?

When my wife was pregnant with our twins, we got a brochure in the ob-gyn's office. Title? "A Good Start: Nutrition During Pregnancy." Copyright? "1988, revised 1992. National Cattlemen's Beef Association."

Forget about no issues of protein deficiency when we get enough calories. Forget about spinach being 40 percent protein by calorie (more than many cuts of beef), and the fact that healthy protein (along with healthy fat and healthy carbohydrates) is in *every* heavy-box food. Forget about the fact that most humans eat too much protein and do best on high-carbohydrate (healthy-carbohydrate, that is) diets.

Forget all that.

Instead, be afraid. Be very afraid.

Living in fear makes it super easy to raise a healthy, vibrant, thriving family. Living in fear sets a darn good example. Right?

RANDY THE MECHANIC

Every so often in my podcast, Randy the Mechanic makes an appearance—kind of an alter ego of sorts. Randy, while being an excellent mechanic, offers not-so-excellent marriage counseling. Crazy, right? Why would anyone go to a mechanic for marriage counseling unless the mechanic was *also* trained in marriage counseling?

Point is to make sure to get advice from practitioners actually trained in the field in which you're looking for advice. People often criticize MDs because they don't get any substantial (if at all) nutrition training in med school. But why should they be criticized for this? It's not part of their job description, not part of medical training, the same way marriage counseling isn't part of Randy's training as a mechanic. Doesn't make them worse doctors, and doesn't make Randy a worse mechanic. They know surgery, pharmaceuticals, and they know them well. Nutrition is not what they're trained to do, so don't hold it against them. At the same time, it's good to know this because if you're looking for nutritional guidance, see a practitioner who is trained in nutrition. With that said, I know of, and know, a bunch of docs who are extremely well versed in nutrition and incredibly knowledgeable. Hope this signals a trend . . .

MOVING ON TO MOVEMENT

Essential to our health and happiness is moving our bodies. Healthy movement lowers stress and gives us a mental/physical kick in the pants.

Here we go.

INTEGRATED EXERCISE

Nutritionally, our bodies work best on food that is natural and whole. Our bodies also work best when we don't stagnate.

But movement doesn't necessarily mean exercise.

What? "Doesn't necessarily mean exercise?"

There is a very specific reason I am writing about movement and not exercise. It's more than semantics. I see a real difference between the two. Exercise isn't necessary, while moving our bodies is. To explain further . . .

Ever notice that wild animals don't exercise? They definitely move around, but not in a jazzercise class and not on a treadmill. Only we humans have to decide to move our bodies for a set period of time and then be able to be largely immobile for most other times. We no longer go over *there* to find food or over *there* to find shelter. Unless our jobs are physical (construction, dance, sports), not a lot of moving around is required in our lives. We travel by machine, sit down a ton, and aren't exactly running away from predators.

Know why it can be difficult getting off the couch to hit a spin class? Because it's optional.

In the healthy-family arena, this presents a challenge. Not only is it a struggle for us (parents) to move our own bodies enough, to get our kids off their butts, we have to compete with iPhones, tablets, video games, and TV shows.

The benefits of movement are well researched and well documented. From the lymph system to blood pressure, from weight management to mood, we are a species that does well when we move.

But contrary to popular belief, it doesn't have to be a huge amount, and certainly doesn't have to be at high intensity.

A few common movement mistakes:

1. People who want to lose weight (or want their children to lose weight) go full-tilt to exercise. They spin the hell out of themselves, run as fast as possible, spend three hours a day at the gym. But diet plays a much bigger role in weight management than movement or exercise—plus, there's a good chance they're pushing too hard and causing themselves undue stress. Remember "run slow"? The no-pain, no-gain philosophy doesn't automatically equal health or happiness.

2. People who exercise for one hour a day and spend the rest of the day completely stagnant, sitting in a chair, staring at a computer screen.

3. People who partake in an exercise they dread . . . If you don't enjoy the exercise you do, find something you do enjoy. FYI, a walk is fantastic exercise. So is a tough spin class if you love it and it makes you feel good. When you enjoy the exercise, you have fun. When you have fun, you're not as stressed. Easy math.

Solution?

Integrate.

I am a huge fan of what I call integrated exercise or integrated movement. I recommend that everyone, regardless of whether they "exercise" every morning (running, biking, swimming, yoga, etc.), integrate movement throughout their day. This might mean a one-minute walk down the hallway at work a few times a day or ten push-ups or squats every hour—or even three push-ups or squats every hour! Getting up from my desk and doing ten lunges takes only thirty seconds. I practice this myself daily. I do run in the morning (because

I love it), and then integrate additional movement throughout my day. It has made a big difference in my energy and fitness. For many of my clients it is their first, and minimally stressful, "in" into daily exercise. No gym membership or equipment purchase required!

Integrated exercise works awesomely for kids, too. Pitching them a super-short walk outside a couple times a day is a completely different animal than telling a child he/she "needs to exercise." Same result, very different delivery.

HAVE YOU FED THE HEAD?

Just as important as how you treat your body is how you treat your mind. Just as important as your child running around outside is your child creating, building, and learning.

Often overlooked in the healthy-living realm is the all-important "mental nutrition." As with physical nutrition (food and movement), there are light-box and heavy-box versions of mental nutrition. And here too, the MOTT applies. We can't all immerse ourselves 100 percent of the time in Tolstoy, know what I'm saying? We also need *St. Elmo's Fire*. (Little-known fact: Tolstoy, under a pseudonym, wrote *St. Elmo's Fire*.)

By way of example, below is a list of lighter- and heavier-box mental "foods." But keep this in mind: The light box list *is* fun, provides much-needed relief, and ain't "bad." In general, however, I argue that lighter-box mental nutrition is best included in your family's life in about the same proportion as light-box meals . . . Here we go:

Lighter-box mental foods:
- Video games
- Social media
- Non–Jane Austen movies
- Non–Jane Austen books
- Non–*Game of Thrones* and non–*Stranger Things* TV shows
- Many articles on news sites (Face it: Past the first paragraph, where you get the gist, is just fluff upon fluff.)

Heavier-box mental foods:
- Novels (like the Jane Austen ones)
- Poetry
- Films (I think we all know the difference between movies and films.)

- Classical music
- Journaling
- Meditation
- Creative pursuits (drawing, painting, dancing, writing, sculpture, collaging, etc.)
- Classes/courses
- Socializing (Actual. With friends/family in person. The way we socialized before we "posted.")

Granted, these lists are just a tad tongue-in-cheek, but a basic way of looking at it is this: escapism versus engagement. Clearly, there are novels that don't challenge us. Fun and awesome, but not challenging. Then, there are novels that move us by the author's sheer use of language, ideas, character, craft, etc. Same goes for movies, TV shows, social media, and the news. I think we all have a pretty good idea of the difference between mindless and mindful entertainment.

My point is that there is a balance to be had with mental nutrition like there is a balance to be had with physical nutrition. A balance of light-box to heavy-box. A way of looking at what you do in your life and making adjustments to change the proportion of light-box to heavy-box if things aren't working the way you'd like them to.

After a rough day at work, some junk food and a fun movie are sometimes just the ticket. However, if these become your MOTT, health and happiness decreases as the stress from which you are escaping increases. We all need the escape once in a while. Once in a while.

It's no small feat setting a good example with mental nutrition. In my house there are plenty of "conversations" (read: battles) with my children on screen time versus outside time, TV shows versus Legos, video games versus reading. I'm in "conversations" (read: battles) with myself about not checking my phone every 3.2 seconds.

As you have no doubt experienced, it takes more energy and attention to read a challenging piece of literature than it does to read a Danielle Steele novel. Both serve their purpose—I'm not advocating doing *only* one or the other. But in the midst of our stressful lives, heavy-box mental food tends to be put on the back burner precisely *because* it takes more effort. Under stress, we're drawn to mindless entertainment just like we're drawn to junk food. Easier for us to zone out, and definitely easier for us to put our kids in front of a television. I get it.

So, with all this talk of heavy-box mental nutrition, you may be thinking, "I'd love to spend time pursuing heavier-box mental nutrition, but I have very limited time, and even more limited energy."

Buckle in.

Here comes the "get 'er done" part of this book. The "making changes *today*" part. The "Yeah, Sid, but what the hell do I do now?" part.

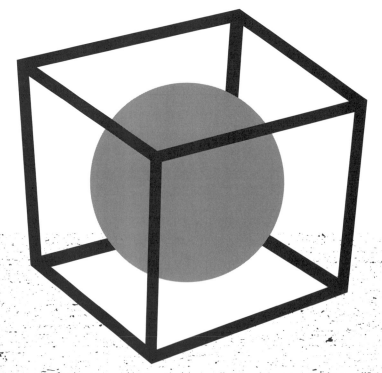

GETTING IT DONE: MY SMALL STEPS APPROACH

This is the part of the book where you put the thinking into action. Where the abstract becomes concrete. Where you get to see your family eat better, move better, be happier, be healthier.

First, what my approach isn't.

It isn't simply breaking your goals into microsteps and doing them one by one. There is way more to it, as you will soon read . . .

Small Stepping starts with learning my system. Becoming a Small Stepper. Then, using the tools, you'll soon learn to create, build, and maintain a Steps List—essentially, a list of new, healthy, and happy-making behaviors that you want to include in your life. Being a Small Stepper takes work but is totally worth it. (Kind of like being married and having children, wouldn't you say?)

The primary reason it is not easy is simply because our lives are full of the things we've already been doing a while. Small Stepping, no matter how awesomely effective I believe it is, is still a new thing to learn. Amid the craziness of today's world, adding anything new is going to be a challenge and a struggle. Once learned, however, my system minimizes the struggle of future "new things." Hang tight . . .

Let's start with tools and tricks to build and maintain a Steps List. The real-life, practical ins and outs of my approach . . .

JUST ANOTHER CRACK IN THE WALL

Most of what we do each day is a series of actions and behaviors that have become just part of our lives. Things we don't think about too much. Brushing our teeth, making our child's breakfast, brewing coffee, driving to work, etc. I call these routines and behaviors the Wall of Behaviors. Anything in the wall has been there for a long time.

Once we have done any new behavior long enough, it is sent to a part of the brain reserved for things we can essentially do automatically, or at least with little or no thought. It is how we don't have to remind ourselves, "Left foot, then right foot, then left foot" when we go for a walk. There was a time, as you know, when we had to learn the skill of walking—the muscle development, the balance, the movement. Only after a sufficient amount of time did walking become automatic and part of our Wall of Behaviors. Same with the thousands of other things we do without having to think too much. And thank goodness for the wall— how could you sing along to the English Beat on your way to work if you still had to pay close attention to every single little thing your hands and feet had to do to drive a car?

Such is the challenge with taking on anything new for you and your family. How to stick with a new behavior long enough to make it a permanent addition to your Wall of Behaviors. How to turn a new behavior into "just something I do" or "just who we are." For example, if you want your family to eat healthier, it doesn't do much good to eat well for a couple days and then call it quits. Eating healthy foods works when "healthy eating" sticks around long enough for it to get into and stay in your wall. No longer new or weird, or stupid. Normal. Or, even more specifically, something you don't really think about.

Like brushing your teeth—part of your wall.

The most common mistake people make when attempting something new is to take on too much, too soon. They don't respect the wall. They try to jam a brand-new, huge chunk into their existing wall. The wall's response? "Yeah, that's not gonna happen."

Take diets . . . Diets don't take the necessary time to introduce new foods/meals in a regulated, minimally stressful way. Just the opposite. They are a 100 percent immersion into new eating habits, new recipes, often new/unfamiliar ingredients, new shopping lists, new kitchen prep, and more. Big, huge chunk o' new behavior forced on the already-existing behaviors (foods someone has been buying, cooking, and eating for years). The wall speaks again: "No room for you here, pal!" Only through the dieter's sheer force of will does he/she get through the seven-day, twenty-one-day, or even three-month period, after which (most likely) his/her old eating habits will come creeping back along with, unfortunately, all the weight lost during the diet.

My Small Steps approach, on the other hand, makes small cracks in the wall. Subtle, little, sneaky cracks that wedge their way in, take hold, and then grow until they, too, become permanent additions. Each Small Step is a new crack. Each Small Step, a new action. Each Small Step, a new behavior.

In other words, it's not about going from your couch to a marathon in four days. It's about starting with a daily five-minute walk that eventually becomes ten, then twenty, then becomes a ten-minute jog, which becomes a thirty-minute jog, and so on until—perhaps not for many months, if not years—the marathon. But here's the hitch . . . A five-minute walk won't work for everyone as a first step, so how do you know what step to start with? What if a five-minute walk is just too much because you haven't taken a walk since Milli Vanilli was a thing?

Which brings me to the two *biggest* misconceptions about my approach:

1. The size of everyone's steps is the same.
2. All Small Steps are very, very small.

Here's the deal . . .

The size of your first step and every step to follow is up to you. One person's Small Step may be too big for another. The size of your step depends on this and this alone: What will create the least amount of stress. Take someone who used to run eight-milers all the time but, with a new job and young children, got out of the routine, and it's been about a year since he has run. Now, he wants to get back to it. For him, a four-mile run a few times per week is an excellent first Small Step. It's easy for him, it's not every day (yet), and, best of all, it's enjoyable. He's on his way . . . . But for someone who has never run, the four-miler is way too much. For that person, that five-minute walk may be just right.

Both small steps. Very different sizes. But both small to *them*.

The step is small if you don't dread it. The step is small if it gets you going with minimal stress. The step is small if it gets you to start doing things you want to do in your life.

This is an approach to your life. It is asking yourself, "What do I want my life to look like, and what am I willing and able to take on that won't burn me out?"

I ask my clients, when they are creating a new step or adjusting an existing one, to ask themselves, "Is this something I could do for the rest of my life?" If they believe they could, it is probably the right-size step at the right time.

Want to start meditating because you read how great it is for stress relief? Does jumping immediately into a forty-five-minute morning meditation seem like a strain? It might be. With children and a job, it'll mean either a big shift in your morning routine or forty-five minutes less sleep. Or both. Yes, with a ton of willpower and effort, not to mention jackhammering out a big ol' chunk in your Wall of Behaviors, you can get that going. Until . . . you start dreading it, skipping it, saying, "To hell with it." Too much, too soon. Willpower gone.

Then the inevitable (but avoidable) outcome: You feel like a failure for not being able to keep it up.

Unfair to you. Not cool.

In contrast, a Small Stepper might say, "I recently read that forty-five minutes of meditation is great, but that is too much to take in right now, given my work schedule, family, and morning routine. So, I'll start with five deep breaths every morning. That'll get the process started, and once meditation is securely in my Wall of Behaviors, I'll build on it until I hit the forty-five minutes." See? No failure.

Action. Success. Happiness.

Less stress.

You can apply my Small Steps approach to food, movement/exercise, creativity, work, parenting, socializing, meditation, and virtually anything else you want to improve or maintain in your life.

Like . . . a healthy and happy family.

UNFAIR TO YOU.
NOT COOL.

HIT A REST STOP ALONG THE WAY

With Small Stepping, you are in charge of both the process and the goal. You are becoming more in control of your life every day.

And sometimes, something interesting happens. For example, during the practice of Small Stepping toward a marathon, you realize that the marathon really isn't your bag. It just feels dang good to run! Your initial step was a five-minute walk. From there, you added (and even subtracted—more on that later) and built, and now, six months in, you can comfortably run a 10K.

You love it. The distance fits. You easily pull it off *and* have plenty of time to get the kids off to school. You run with your buddies on the weekends, and you've lost weight, have more energy, and find yourself exploring other areas to Small Step into. All great stuff, but you realize that the original goal of the marathon has lost a little pizazz. Thing is, you've got other fish to fry now that you didn't have six months ago, so you blow off the marathon, stick with 10Ks, and are a happier person for it.

Your life. Your goals.

Change 'em, keep 'em. Up to you.

Life not only goes on without the marathon, you also feel more powerful because you are taking charge of your life.

And who knows? When the kids are old enough to drive and you have extra time on your hands, you might put a marathon back on the table.

Same goes for food. You won't find what works for you by following a diet. No rest stops to assess along the way. Just the plan/chart, and you're following it. But maybe . . . day twelve isn't you. It's *not* your MOTT, and it isn't helping you find out what is. The only way to find out? Introduce healthy food in a low-stress way (your own custom version of little by little) and then build until you hit a good balance. A balance that works for you and your family. Boom. You nailed it.

Okay, we're done.

That is the gist of my Small Steps approach.

Pint-sized version: Find out who you truly are, what you stand for (remember the first task?), areas you want to change to get you closer to who you truly are, then . . . figure out appropriately sized steps that get the ball rolling.

Approaching your life this way does yield huge transformation. Just not overnight. Thank goodness.

Now, on to the nuts and bolts of effectively stepping into new behaviors.

LET'S GET MARRIED

G reat trick of the Small Stepper's trade . . .

One way to Small Step with your family into a new, healthy behavior is to utilize your existing Wall of Behaviors. You pick one of the routines in your life and use it as an anchor for one of your steps. In other words, you marry the new behavior to one that is already in the wall. To illustrate this, here are some parent hypotheticals.

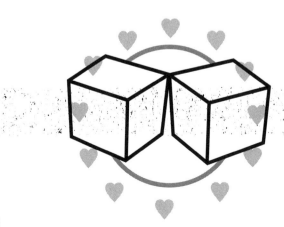

PARENT HYPOTHETICAL #1

You want to meditate in the morning because you think it will help set a better tone for the day. Let's just say you've been a little edgy around the kids and need a little more calm, focus, and overall chill. So . . . you think about it and decide that four deep breaths is your Small Step. "Okay," you say, "let's frickin' do this!"

Four days later, you realize you haven't done the breaths. Not once. What the heck? It's only four deep breaths, for crying out loud. Thirty seconds, tops! "I should be able to pull this off," you say.

Solution: Find an existing behavior to anchor the deep-breaths step to. One that you basically do without thinking, like brushing your teeth. Remember when you were a child, your parents had to remind you time and time again to brush your teeth? Eventually, it became part of your wall, so that now you get up every morning, shuffle into the bathroom half-asleep, and brush away. Autopilot . . . And the perfect behavior to marry your deep-breaths step to.

Here's what you do: Write a little note that says "Deep breaths" and tape it to either your mirror or the toothbrush itself. See what happens. Spoiler alert: Tomorrow morning, you will wander half-asleep into the bathroom like always, but this time, as you grab for the brush, you'll see the note and take your deep breaths. Meditation? Done.

Boom.

"But, Sid! Four deep breaths doesn't do squat! Guru Richie Rich said meditation is forty-five minutes on a pillow in front of a candle and a Buddha statue, or in a cave in the Himalayas, assuming an unenlightened person brings me food and stuff to build a fire with."

First of all, no. Second of all, we're not there yet.

The four-deep-breaths step is the starting point. The first of possibly many steps. The crack in the Wall of Behaviors. It may eventually grow to forty-five minutes. Or not. Either way, you're making moves. You're adding in a healthy behavior. You're kicking ass. Take the breaths, and then pat yourself on the back.

A SIDEBAR (JUST BETWEEN YOU AND ME)

You will be amazed at how difficult even the seemingly smallest of Small Steps can be. Most of my clients start with a step of texting me first thing in the morning a simple, one-word message (like "Up" or "Awake"). This text serves as a first-thought-before-the-craziness—a reminder of the work they're doing. It should be easy, right? It only takes four seconds . . . However, a fair number have a tough time with this step. They wake up each morning, and their lives (and Wall of Behaviors) come rushing in. Kids, lunches, work stress, washing dishes, brushing teeth. Rushing in. That's been their morning for years. So, even though it takes only four seconds, the text is a new behavior that requires additional effort and attention.

Conclusion? Part of the Small Steps process. Nothing to sweat. Something to solve with the Small Stepper's bag of tools and tricks.

Okay, back to it—and, hey . . . glad we had this little talk.

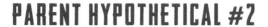

PARENT HYPOTHETICAL #2

You want to spend more time with your friends. You've been so frickin' busy with work and family that you haven't even been able to eke out a phone conversation, much less a cup of coffee, with your pal. You want to do this because you miss it, it makes you feel better, and having this in your life makes you a happier parent. Let's face it, you miss Cindy. I mean, she's one in a million.

The last time you saw her, you said, "We should really do this more often!" And yet, in a blink of an eye, six months have gone by since you've seen her.

Solution: You settle on a Small Step for time with Cindy (with her input, hopefully), then look for an existing behavior to marry it to. Hmmm. How about grocery shopping? You do it anyways. You do it on Sundays. You spend thirty minutes to an hour at the grocery store. Every week.

Here's what you do: Call Cindy, who, in a surprising turn, shops for groceries, too. Pitch the idea that since you both shop for groceries, why not shop at the same time, same day, same place? This Sunday, you meet her at the market. You do your shopping together. Literally walk down the aisles together, chatting along the way. Then, for a few minutes post-checkout, you have a sit-down. Maybe even a cup of coffee and a chat. (Your market doesn't sell hot coffee? What kind of insane store are you frequenting that doesn't sell brewed coffee?!?)

Five minutes is all you can manage for the sit-down? Better than nothing, wouldn't you say? And just the starting point. Cindy is back. You have a little jolt of fun, of support, of socializing. You've stepped out of your bubble, and even though it is just a few minutes, it some-how makes a difference in your life. And then . . . after a few weeks, you make plans to go out to dinner one night a month, perhaps. Who knows? But . . . you've stopped your life from passing you by.

Result: You come home to the family in a better, happier state. The socializing enhances your life and even makes the grocery shopping more fun. Happier you, happier parent.

TECHNOLOGY: BAD!

Except no, technology is not bad. It's how we use it. It's like the old adage: Laser-tag guns don't fake-kill people, fourteen-year-olds with laser-tag guns fake-kill people.

Technology can be a Small Stepper's BFF. Remember the first-thing-in-the-morning texting step? That's using technology to help steal a moment.

To-do lists and calendars go hand-in-hand with smartphones. Sure, they are used for mundane things like meetings, grocery lists, and doctor's appointments, but they work great for Small Steps, too. Simply create a separate list for your Small Steps.

Remember my integrated exercise? I use an app that shoots me an integrated exercise reminder on the hour during the day. (See the Resources section.) I've been doing this for a couple years, and this app is still incredibly useful. Like most people, my days get super busy. Having this reminder go off is like having someone tap me on the shoulder every hour to say, "Hey, drop down and do a few push-ups—you'll feel better for it." We have the phones in our darn pockets anyway. Why not use them to get the real us out of the shadows?

Onward and upward.

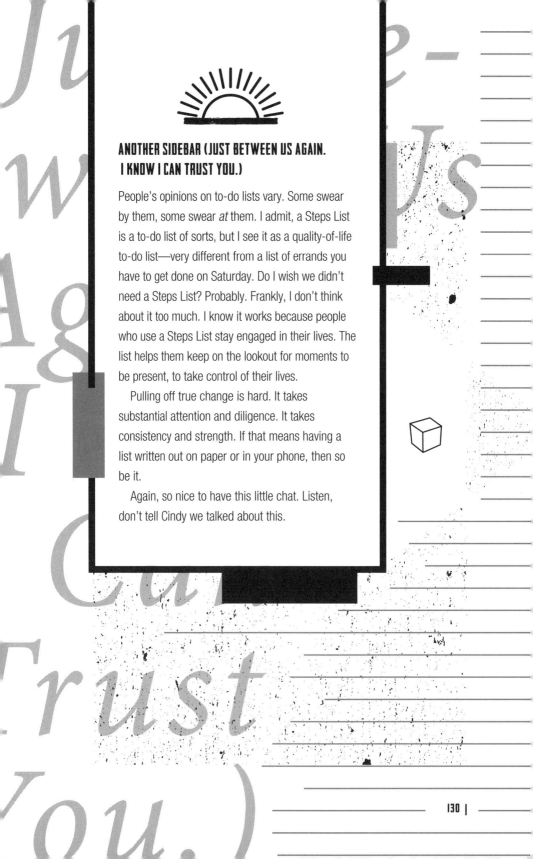

ANOTHER SIDEBAR (JUST BETWEEN US AGAIN. I KNOW I CAN TRUST YOU.)

People's opinions on to-do lists vary. Some swear by them, some swear *at* them. I admit, a Steps List is a to-do list of sorts, but I see it as a quality-of-life to-do list—very different from a list of errands you have to get done on Saturday. Do I wish we didn't need a Steps List? Probably. Frankly, I don't think about it too much. I know it works because people who use a Steps List stay engaged in their lives. The list helps them keep on the lookout for moments to be present, to take control of their lives.

Pulling off true change is hard. It takes substantial attention and diligence. It takes consistency and strength. If that means having a list written out on paper or in your phone, then so be it.

Again, so nice to have this little chat. Listen, don't tell Cindy we talked about this.

THE FRIENDS-AND-FAMILY PLAN

After two hugely effective tools to help build and maintain a Steps List, marrying steps and using technology, there is a third and equally effective tool: friends and family.

In *Approaching the Natural*, I wrote about the pros and cons of Weight Watchers (or at least the old-school, 1970s version). Pros? Definitely the social aspect. Sharing your experiences with others, and offering and receiving support from peers. Cons? French fries = 6 points. On what planet do French fries only get 6 points? Not cool, Weight Watchers.

Having a pal and/or family member and/or coworker who is either coming along for the ride with their own Steps List or just having your back to help you with yours is invaluable.

Even a non–Small Stepping spouse/partner will likely be game to lend a helping hand to remind you of your steps.

Friends might even be game to try out what you're doing just for kicks. Instead of doing a diet together, try Small Stepping. Your lists will be different, but the approach will be the same. In fact, you might ask Cindy if she'd help you out with your list. You'll see her at the grocery store on Sunday.

Oh, and tell her hi from me. Cindy is awesome.

Oh, and one more thing while we're on the subject: Don't forget to offer your own support for a pal on his/her own trek (Small Steps or otherwise). It feels good to help someone in this way and can be a learning process for you—more to learn about what does and doesn't work.

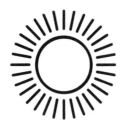

ANOTHER SIDEBAR

Little, but fair, warning . . . When you talk to others about changes you make in your life, they might feel threatened and/or judged. As if the Small Steps you're taking for yourself and your family are saying something about them. So . . . make sure that, if/when you ask folks to help you be accountable to your list, you make it clear this isn't about them. It really isn't. Simply tell them it's important to you and you could really use their help.

I have worked with clients whose spouses, while wanting absolutely nothing to do with healthy living, are more than happy to offer support and encouragement. If this is you, be satisfied with that. Don't expect them to change or ask them to. Focus on your own practice, improve the example you are setting, and you never know what might happen.

SUBTRACTION IS ADDITION

We hate going backward. If we step to the point where we easily run four-milers, the thought of running less feels like we're backtracking. Not doing enough. But hold on a sec . . .

Sometimes our lives change—new job, new commute, new town—and that four-miler may be tough to pull off. It becomes a time crunch, a stress to fit in, while running just a couple miles would work a lot better, except we think it's "not enough."

I see things differently.

Remember, the steps are there because they are minimally stressful and easy to pull off. As a Small Stepper, you only increase a step (from four breaths to five breaths) when you are ready for the increase and not super stressed by it.

But what if life *does* change, and that previously low-stress step becomes unmanageable?

Solution? You decrease the step.

Four miles goes down to two. Ten deep breaths goes down to five. Twenty minutes of journaling goes down to seven.

It looks like you're doing less. It feels like you're regressing. Know what you are really doing?

Succeeding.

Success: Taking good care of yourself. Being in charge. Doing what it takes to decrease your overall stress because it is good for you and your family.

Continuing to push forward in spite of significant stress and in the name of forward momentum means your Steps List has taken charge of you, not the other way around. The list has become a lot like a diet—something you unquestioningly follow with little or no regard for the effect it has on your life.

Decreasing steps to keep you from burning out, to keep your list active, to keep you engaged in your life, really is *adding* to the quality of your life. For a Small Stepper, sometimes subtraction is addition.

THE FAMILY LIST

This book is called *Raising Healthy Parents* because when it comes to healthy, less-stressed families, it is mostly about the parents.

Which means, building *your* own Steps List is primo. Maintaining it, adding to it, living it.

But what about the rest of the family?

To make changes specific to your family, you can go either of these ways:

1. Include family-directed steps on YOUR list:
   a. Read to my children for five minutes per day. (**Explanation:** You had a plan to read for an hour every day but realized it was too much because you haven't read for, well, months. Five minutes is doable and gets the act on your radar. Boom.)
   b. Play one game with my children per weekend. (**Explanation:** No matter what your grand plans are for your weekends, they get miraculously filled up with laundry, cleaning, and errands. But one game is doable and doesn't become just another dreaded task to get through. Quality over quantity, and you still have time to fluff and fold.)
2. Create a Family List, and craft it *with* your family:
   a. One family adventure per weekend. (**Explanation:** An adventure can be whatever you want it to be—going

somewhere you've never been, like a store, park, building, museum—or any activity you have never done, even a drive down a street you have never seen. Ask your children for ideas. Most kids are more than ready for an adventure, no matter how small.)

b. Three family meals per week. (**Explanation:** Family meals are the perfect "married" step. You eat anyway, so marry the meal with quality family time. Because of my life and my work, family meals take a concerted effort. Totally worth it.)

c. One family night per week. (**Explanation:** This can be tough depending on the age of your children and/or your schedule, so this step could also be one family night every two weeks or even once a month. Anything is better than nothing. And . . . family night can be anything—out to dinner, to a movie, with extended family. At my house, it is making a meal together and renting a movie. Pretty simple, totally affordable, and a highlight of the week.)

FUN WITHOUT FOOD? WTF?

Yes. It exists. Fun without food. And it may surprise you to know that it is possible to watch a movie without eating or drinking anything. Who knew?

Fact is, we opened a Pandora's box when we learned to manipulate food to such a degree that it gets us high. And because this get-us-high food is so darn accessible (and the cheapest game in town), it is super easy to "enhance" pretty much any experience with it. Movie *with* popcorn, movie *with* candy. And yet . . . it is worth experimenting with nonfood fun. A walk with the family, listening to music, and yes, even watching a movie without food. Not to restrict, but to grab even more fulfillment from the people you are with.

I have worked with many clients for whom food is their major tool for stress relief. Not exactly uncommon. I will often recommend they build in steps of nonfood fun in addition to their food fun. This could be something like a five-minute family walk outside before sitting down to a meal. One client would listen to music for a few minutes before dinner. Result? He found himself eating less, eating healthier, and enjoying the meal even more, just by creating a moment of nonfood joy. Who doesn't have five minutes?

Everyone has five minutes.

HELD IN THE HIGHEST ESTEEM

Each time we accomplish something, we add a little notch in the belt of self-confidence and self-esteem. Reaching goals strengthens us and positively affects virtually every other part of our lives. Conversely, not accomplishing, not reaching our goals, affects us negatively.

Enter Small Steps.

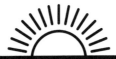

SIDEBAR: SMALL STEPS FOR SMALL PEOPLE

Like parents, children can very quickly feel overwhelmed. We can help them with this by breaking down their to-do's into manageable, minimally stressful steps. For instance, teaching them to ease into their schoolwork (book reports, essays, papers in general) teaches them more effective study tools (i.e., not to procrastinate) and lowers *their* overall stress.

Unfortunately, I didn't learn this until my senior year of college, but when I did, it paid off big-time. As a philosophy major, my work was almost entirely about papers (multiple-choice tests and philosophy don't mix well). In my last year of school, I began working on papers the very same day they were assigned and working on them a little bit each day. My results? Dean's honors list, better learning, no all-nighters, and far less stress. Teaching young children these tools sets them up for greater success. They learn to work harder, work better, and, best of all, manage their own stress.

You can teach your children to apply this approach with anything from spelling tests (e.g., focus on four words per day) to piano practice (e.g., start with ten minutes a day), and chores (e.g., clean the room for five minutes per day instead of waiting until it gets so bad, it takes hours). By making the step small, your child won't fight you on it. And often, by just getting them started on the task, they'll end up putting in more time than originally planned.

Bonus: Less stress for them means less stress for you. Happier household.

Each Small Step is a goal.

Completing each Small Step is an accomplishment. Maybe not newsworthy. Probably not even tell-your-friend worthy. But, *you* know.

Approaching your life as a Small Stepper is like being in daily accomplishment training. Forever. You get very used to taking action and taking control of your life. You get very used to feeling confident in your ability to live life on your terms.

Not that marathons and diets aren't goals as well. They are. When you cross the finish line or complete the twenty-one-day diet, you feel great because of what you accomplished. But both the marathon and the diet are down-the-line goals. Get-to-the-end goals.

Small Stepping is in addition to these types of goals. Small Stepping is day-to-day, and even moment-to-moment. You set and accomplish goals all the time, and each time, it feels good. No waiting for the finish line.

So, while you're clocking off the mileage every morning on your way to race day, your Steps List is right there, too. Showing you how to take control of your entire life, for the rest of your life.

Self-confidence and self-esteem come with work and struggle. They come with accomplishment and achievement. They come with learning how to prevent the craziness of the world from getting the best of you.

This is what you bring to your family. This rubs off on your spouse and your children. Message: We can do this. We can do better. We can grow, improve, and evolve. Instead of setting massive and unattainable goals that increase our chances of failure (e.g., starting today, we are 100 percent changing what we eat!), we set attainable, minimally stressful goals and set ourselves up for success every day.

Teach your child to work on his/her report five minutes per day—not to wait until the very last minute. And note the difference in your child's stress, how his/her mood is each day after completing the five minutes. Daily accomplishment. Learning to work, learning self-care—not just by doing a better job on the report, but by minimizing the stress of the process.

READY, SET, GO

I'm going to assume you are game to use Small Steps to help your family thrive. But it probably means a conversation with the troops: A "Here's a-what we're gonna do, everyone."

Communicating change is a tricky business. Changing the food you eat? Dang.

How do you set out the plan in a way that doesn't cause rebellion or a freakout?

It takes care and attention, much like the change itself.

I think you'd agree that "Because I said so" explanations are best minimized. Not that I don't pull them out once in a while. There's definitely a time and a place—"Get out of the street!" "Why?" "Because I said so!" (followed by a quiet, exasperated "Jiminy Christmas" to myself). The long-term nature of this approach allows parents to take their time in the way they communicate it.

So, what do you say to them?

KIDS UNDERSTAND
THE DARNEDEST THINGS

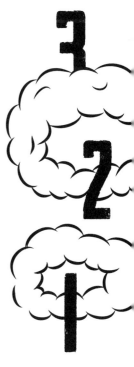

I believe children understand far more than we give them credit for, but it is incumbent on us to take care with the way we explain things. This could not be more relevant than with Small Stepping.

First, frame these steps for what they truly are: goals and actions to improve things at home, to make everyone happier. This goes a long way with children.

In other words, instead of, "We are not going to eat any more junk food, so we can all lose weight," how about, "We are going to start eating healthier food more often, because we like to run around, play with friends, and go on trips." The first, while technically true, doesn't paint the whole picture.

When I teach nutrition/healthy-living classes, I begin with the question "Why eat healthy?" What people don't know is that every single time I flash that question on the screen, I cringe. And it's my frickin' slide, for crying out loud. I cringe because on the surface, the question seems trite and obvious. But . . . it's a deeper question when you apply just a little more thought to it.

Typical responses are "to lose weight" or "to decrease my chances of cancer/diabetes/heart disease, etc." or "to decrease inflammation in my body." All fine, except that isn't *actually* why they are taking a class on nutrition and healthy living. Here's why: Deep down, they want to feel alive, not just stay alive. There is a huge divide between feeling alive and being alive. Huge. Losing weight is just one stop on our way to feeling vibrant and alive. (There are plenty of thin yet unhealthy people.) We want to have the energy to do the things we want to do. We want to be happy. Nutrition and exercise are excellent tools to get us there, but they are only tools.

So, too, with parents. So, too, with children. So, too, with families. Getting children outside to play isn't about exercise. It's about teaching them the tools to live well. Think about it this way, and the fruit smoothie becomes as much a treat as the Jolly Frickin' Rancher. The better we communicate that, the easier it is to make changes.

If your children are old enough to have a conversation, they can grasp a fair amount of why you are embarking on the changes represented on your Steps List. There is no need for a formal, heavy, serious family sit-down. Because of the long-term nature of this approach, communication can trickle in before and during the changes.

SAMPLE SMALL STEP AND "THE WHY"

SAMPLE STEP Ten minutes of quality family time every Saturday and Sunday (either a walk, a board game, or an art project).

THE WHY "Because it's so much fun to spend time with you! All of us being together is super fun, right? So, what do you feel like doing? A walk, a game, draw some pictures?"

ENROLL IN THE ROLE

The "What do you feel like doing?" is the key. Involve your children in the steps. Ask them for their help, ask them for their input, even ask them for advice.

"Hey, [insert hipster child name here—Dylan?], can you help me pick out some healthy food at the market today?" Or, "Hey Sophia/Sophie/Hannah, what do you think—grilled asparagus or sautéed zucchini with our dinner tonight?" or, "I'm tired. Do you think a short walk would get me going?"

Works great for meals. More on this in the upcoming recipe/meal section, but create-your-own-type meals go a long way. You empower your child by making them an active participant, but in an environment where as a parent, you determine the options. In other words, "Asparagus or zucchini?" *not* "Asparagus or Twinkie?" Engaging them in the process also inspires questions and conversations around healthy living. Way more subtle and positive than presenting a list of "we now only eat these foods from now on." Asking your child to help you pick out heavy-box foods at the market starts a relaxed, informal convo about which foods are healthy and why. No need to have the *entire*, in-depth conversation on aisle 7. Discussing one or two foods at a time is a great start. Remember, ease in. It makes the change almost unnoticeable.

MAKE THE ABNORMAL NORMAL

In my house, the discussion of college is never a "So, you think you might wanna, you know, maybe, eventually—and you know it's totally up to you, but maybe you might wanna—go to college?"

Rather, the discussion isn't much of a discussion at all. The subject of college is expressed in throwaway comments, assumptions, and informal references. Such as "Your mom and I had an awesome time at college. You guys will love it." Or, "After college, you might want to travel a bit before you start working."

Could all three of my children decide to skip college? Of course. But we want them to see college as normal. Not something extra, special, or crazy/unattainable. Just something you do. Grammar school, high school, college, and postgrad (if that floats their boat). When it sounds normal, it sounds less "big."

Same goes for healthy eating. All three of my children could grow up and choose to eat only SpaghettiOs. Small Stepping into healthy eating draws much less attention to heavy-box foods than a massive, all-at-once change. Make living healthy *not* that big of a deal, and, well, it's not that big of a deal.

Any new thing you introduce is abnormal until, with enough time and consistency, it becomes normal.

Time. Consistency.

DON'T FORGET TO BRUSH YOUR TEETH AND WASH YOUR BRAIN

P arents brainwashing their children. Good, or bad?

Neither.

Know why?

Because it happens whether you like or not. You are the example for your children whether you are a good example or a bad example. They're buying what you're selling.

So . . .

I say go bigger. Brainwash the crap out of your children. Just be a kick-ass brainwasher. Be *more* involved in the process. Not less. Play the "I'll let my children make their own choices about what they eat" game, and the example you set is a parent who can't bother to—or, worse, is afraid to—instill healthy habits.

Be more aware of what you're dishing out, because your children are listening and watching ALL the time, whether you like it or not.

This may happen (and it did to me): You send your children to school with a lunch filled with glorious heavy-box foods—one that is in stark contrast to the "normal" string-cheese, hardboiled-egg, gold-fish-cracker, cheese-sandwich-on-white-bread lunches—and someone comments that you are brainwashing your child.

How do you respond?

"Yep."

WAIT, DON'T TALK WEIGHT

As I wrote previously, I view healthy weight as but one side effect of health. Beyond that, I argue that nobody actually wants to lose weight. What they want is to feel good, look good, have more energy and more vitality. Conversation about weight falls way short. Ain't the real goal. For this reason, I steer people away from any talk of weight. Irrelevant to my work. I don't help people lose weight. I help them gain health.

When it comes to overweight children, you should talk about their weight this many times:

Zero.

And make sure that no steps on your list even rhyme with "weight loss." Instead, *add in* heavier-box foods, *add in* movement, *add in* quality family time.

Communicate the truth. The family really is Small Stepping to feel better and happier. As a parent, *you* understand that including more heavy-box foods and movement will lead to healthy weight, but it ain't the "thing," so don't make it the "thing."

Long-term result? Your child grows into an adult who focuses on self-care, on adding in, on self-nourishing. An adult who doesn't yo-yo diet. Ever.

TO CHOOSE, OR NOT TO CHOOSE

emember way, way back in this book, when we were just getting to know each other, I wrote about how we shouldn't forget we are animals? My point is that as animals, our needs are really quite simple. If we cut through the crap, if we block out all the media, advertising, and entertainment just for a moment, we realize we don't need all that much to be happy and healthy.

For instance, animals in nature do not grapple with food the way we do. They don't wander around the forest, indecisive about what to eat for their next meal: "Hmmm, Mexican or Italian?" They don't feel the pang of "Man, I really want that third cookie, but I *shouldn't*."

Humans do. We grapple, wring our hands, attend classes and lectures, and talk about how darn hard it is to eat healthy. With most of us having an absolutely insane selection of heavy-box foods at our disposal, our species just can't get healthier. The healthy food is there, and we ain't taking advantage of it.

Hmmm . . . ever wonder why that is?

Here's why: We *also* have an insane selection of light-box fast food and junk food.

When you think about it, we basically have access to a ton of frickin' food in general, healthy or unhealthy, and the sheer weight of that choice is on our shoulders. It is up to us to choose. Ironically, the number of choices we have make choosing all that much harder.

Next time you walk into a grocery store, just pause for a moment and take in the selections at your fingertips. Then, notice the proportion of packaged/bottled/manufactured food to naked plants on the shelf. Staggering. The reason for the larger proportion of packaged foods?

They're invented with the sole purpose of lighting our heads on fire. They're technologically altered to become more drug than food. Cap'n Crunch may be fortified with a small handful of vitamins and minerals, but let's be clear—it wasn't my sophomore-year-at-college, two-in-the-morning go-to "food" because it would supply me with sufficient levels of B6 and zinc.

We are up against this reality when we make the decision that it's time for our families to eat healthier.

Fear not. I have a solution. And it ain't necessarily to never experience the life- and mind-altering Cap'n Crunch.

Here's what I suggest: Minimize choice in your home. Make your home the home base. The sanctuary. The battle-free zone. A "food as drug"-free environment.

In other words, stock your house with awesomeness, with real, mostly natural, delicious, healthy food so you get a break from all the choice and struggle that comes with attempting health in a massively unhealthy world.

Reasons why this works:

1. If you don't have a bunch of light-box foods in the house, you decrease battles with your children. So much easier to say, "We don't have that" than "You can't have that." Then, make a kick-ass-tasting heavy-box meal. Children may rebel now and then, but ultimately, if they're hungry, they'll eat. And when they do, you'll be there with food that will nourish. They'll adjust very quickly and enjoy it. Regardless, someone's gotta have their backs.

2. Making your home more of a choiceless environment means you don't have to sweat the parties or other social engagements where lighter-box foods abound. Your

MOTT is secure. Remember, one-offs don't make much difference.

3. Having less food choice at home means less conflict for you individually. (Independent of your child. I know, shocking concept.) You come home from work craving ice cream, but if it's not in the freezer, chances are slim you are leaving your family to go back out and get some. More likely, you'll probably come to and realize you didn't really want it in the first place, and instead you look for a better solution to relieve the stress of the bad day at work.

4. Your home becomes a de facto habit builder. You eat healthier at home because it is what's there. The more often you eat it, the better it tastes. Healthy eating becomes normal faster.

5. Less choice in the home means less chance of you doing something you (the first-task you) does not want to do. Less regret, less guilt, less shame. Three things we could all do without.

RECIPES AND SA

MPLE MEAL PLANS

RECIPES AND SA

MPLE MEAL PLANS

RECIPES AND SA

MPLE MEAL PLANS

Small Steppers note:

Wherever possible, make double

batches for freezing!

MEALTIME

O kay. What follows is a closer (nay, "refreshing") look at food, but in a real-life, in-the-house, what-the-heck-do-I-do-for-dinner kind of way.

The point here is *not* to overwhelm you with a ton of recipes (there are thousands of great cookbooks out there, if that's your bag), but to sell you on a simple idea:

Minimize the overall time spent on food (shopping, prepping, cooking, thinking about, planning), and buy more time for yourself and your family.

Hear me out.

DIFFICULT, SHMIFFICULT

C ontrary to popular belief (popular belief often being as nutty nut nut as conventional wisdom), eating healthy is *not* difficult. Eating healthy does not take more time. Anyone who tells you otherwise is either selling something or trying to make himself feel better about his own food choices.

My wife and I have three children. We both work full time. Yet our family eats very healthily most of the time. Are we superheroes? No . . . though . . . in the early days of our marriage, we'd dress up as—wait. Did I just write that?

Contrary to conventional wisdom, we are not superheroes. We're parents raising families, just like you. We spend no more time in the kitchen than any average family. We do breakfast, lunch, snacks, and dinner just like everyone else. Well, almost.

We do healthy versions of all those meals, and we've been doing it a while.

At the time we transitioned, it was harder. We learned new recipes, new ingredients, new nutritional information. It was harder because, in the beginning, any change takes effort and attention. Doing anything differently means having to pay attention to it until it becomes your new normal. Comes with the territory. The question is whether it is worth the short-term effort, the getting over the hump, or not. If it's worth it, you'll stick with it long enough for it to become routine. But don't dismiss out of hand something as important as feeding your family well, because it'll be a little harder before it gets easy.

Between you and me? Even if healthy eating never got easier for us, we'd *still* frickin' do it.

TIPS AND TRICKS

C hanging foods overnight can be really unpleasant, but rest assured, your family's taste buds will come along for the ride. After a matter of weeks, they will adjust to new flavors and enjoy them. However, these tips and tricks will help shuttle your family through the transition a little easier.

1. **The Great Sneak Approach.** While I advocate for open communication with your children about the why of healthy living, being a bit of a sneak goes a long way.
   a. Got Un-Milk? A cow's-breast milk product (milk, cheese, yogurt, sour cream) has no business in the human body—child or adult. I am asthma-free because I realized that fact many years ago and made

the change. (It was not a fluke. See the Resources section.) When my children finished breastfeeding from my human wife (felt the need to clarify), they were, well, done with breastfeeding for good. But for many families, pouring a child a glass of milk with dinner is a routine. If that's you, try sneaking in a little nondairy (soy, almond, hemp, rice) milk with the cow's milk to begin the weaning process. Then, over time, shift the proportion of nondairy milk to cow's milk until the glass of "milk" no longer has breast milk in it. On the cheese front . . . some nondairy cheeses are not healthy but still a step up from cow's-milk cheese. Adjusting the proportions with cheese works well, too—start with half cow's-milk cheddar and half nondairy cheddar, and then adjust from there.

Side note: There is nothing to fear with soy. See the Resources section for recommended reading, including books that debunk the myths. It's astounding the amount of misinformation out there on soy. Lots of fear, and you know how I feel about fear.

b. The Meatball-Disappearing Act. Let's say your child loves meatballs. I mean, *loves* 'em. Take them away tomorrow, and you'll have a mutiny on your hands. But . . . sneak/mix in some finely chopped veggies (broccoli, zucchini, spinach, kale) to the meatballs during prep, and you've upped the micronutrients in the meal. Cover it with sauce, and it'll go down unnoticed. However, make sure to check out the awesome lentil "meatball" recipe that follows.

2. **Like Water for Oil.** Oils (olive, corn, canola, coconut, etc.)

are super high in calories and definitely light-box. Using even a few tablespoons to sauté your veggies makes the meal mostly olive oil. (Calorically . . . remember caloric concentration? Nice work.) Minimizing or avoiding oil is an easy way to up the proportion of heavy-box to light-box calories. Here are a couple of tricks . . .

    a. When sautéing onions and garlic, vegetable broth gets the job done, but you can also try this: Heat up your pan *without* oil and, once it's hot, add the oil. Using oven mitts, pick up the pan and swirl the oil around until the pan is well coated. (Since the pan is hot, the oil will move around easily.) Then dump out any excess oil, which will leave only a very thin layer in the pan. You've just significantly reduced the overall light-box calories!

    b. For veggies in general, braise them in veggie stock/broth instead of sautéing in oil. Still tastes great—spice/flavor as you would normally.

    c. Sauce first, ask questions later. When preparing pasta, instead of throwing in a bunch of olive oil into the drained pasta, add in the sauce. It'll keep the pasta from sticking, but with a fraction of the oil (especially if you're using a low-oil or no-oil sauce—like the alfredo sauce in the recipe/meal ideas section).

3. **The "Salads Rule" Rule.** In my house, a salad comes on every dinner plate. It's a given. We don't ask, "Do you want a salad?" We ask "What dressing do you want?" It's normal, it's awesome, and we even include salads with our weekend/not-as-healthy/treat meals. Great first Small Steps are stalks of celery, sliced carrots, tomato slices, or cucumber sticks, and then eventually building to a salad.

4. **A Bowl Cut.** Two of my three children love bowls—basically, a bunch of stuff thrown together in a bowl with a sauce (teriyaki, cashew ranch dressing, salsa, or a combo). Pastas, veggie sautés, beans, quinoa put into a bowl with cut veggies and lettuce, then mixed around. Easy to throw together, and let your children choose their own sauces!

REGULARITY, UNDERLINED

Went with the underline. Bringing out the big guns.

I hear from more and more people that they feel overwhelmed by meal planning, prep, shopping, and cooking every day. On top of everything else, having to come up with new meal ideas every week, and then having to learn new recipes, takes a huge amount of time.

If that describes you, try this on for size:

Plan out a standard weekly meal plan that remains the same week to week. Meaning, you have a regular Monday meal, a regular Tuesday

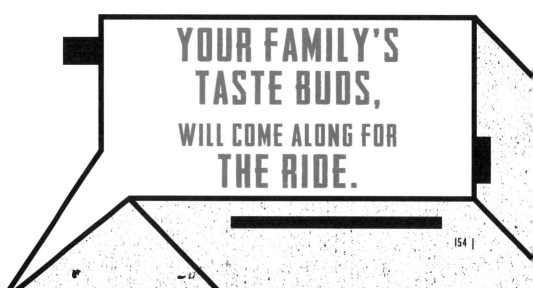

YOUR FAMILY'S TASTE BUDS, WILL COME ALONG FOR THE RIDE.

meal, a regular Wednesday meal, and so on. My family has a regular Monday-through-Friday plan that pretty much stays the same. Saturday and Sunday vary because we have more time to cook, and enjoy it when we do.

Creating a regular week-to-week plan means:

- Shopping gets quicker and easier. By repeating recipes each week, you learn exactly where to find the ingredients at the grocery store, making your shopping trips a ton faster. More time saved to read *Pride and Prejudice*. My local co-op market makes fun of me because I'm their fastest shopper. I'm usually in and out of there in five to seven minutes.
- Preparing and cooking get quicker and easier. After only a few weeks of making your regular list, you'll effortlessly bang out the recipes. Best part is that prep becomes so easy, it becomes more of a hangout time. Time you can spend talking to your children, assisting with homework, or hanging out with your spouse. Less attention on food, more attention freed up for other things.

WHY NO MORE THAN 15 MEALS? BECAUSE I SAID SO.

I am including the fifteen recipes/meal ideas that follow as examples of easy heavy-box meals your family will dig. Recipes that could be contenders for your MOTT. Try them out. See what the family thinks. Then, choose four or five of their/your favorites to use as your regulars. The bonus? Many of the recipes make great leftovers for the next day's school lunches. Even more time saved.

By way of example, here is what the Garza-Hillman week looks like on the dinner front . . .

EVERY MONDAY: VEGGIE-BURGER TOSTADAS
EVERY TUESDAY: TOFU/BROCCOLINI PASTA
EVERY WEDNESDAY: TACO NIGHT
EVERY THURSDAY: POTATO NIGHT
EVERY FRIDAY: I work late at the wellness center, so my wife and kids have dinner with my in-laws, who live next door. To be clear, they invite "us" for dinner on the night I can't make it. Apparently, they don't like me. So weird—I mean, what's not to like?

▢ QUICK REMINDER

We have made these dishes so many times, we can do them in our sleep. We spend zero time on meal planning and shopping lists. We know what to buy and where to get everything. Dialed in.

Last point—if one of your regular recipes gets old after a while, simply switch it out for a new "regular" and get rolling again. After a few weeks, you'll get up to speed with it.

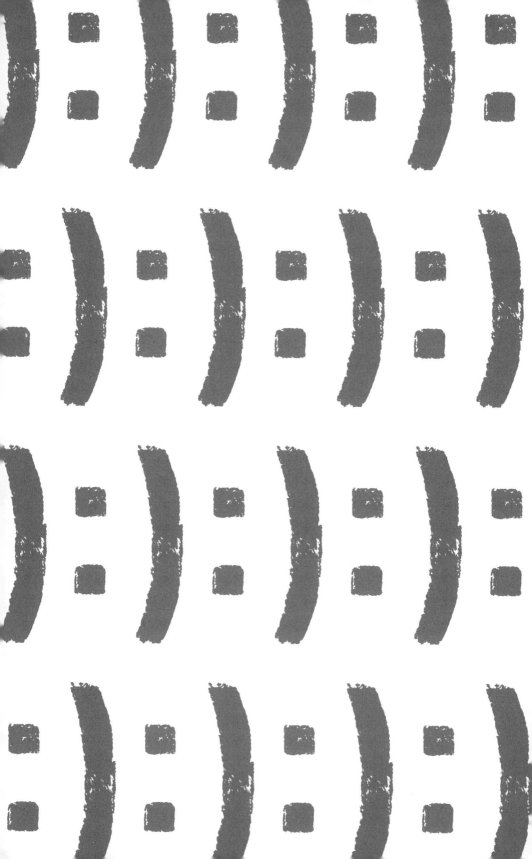

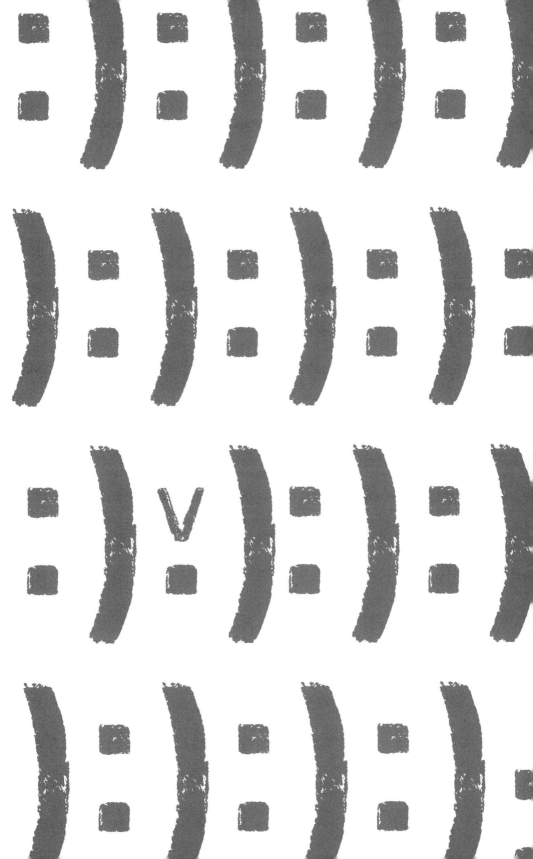

CAULIFLOWER BISQUE

This is an easy and awesome soup. You cook it with the entire sprig of thyme. During the cooking, the thyme leaves will fall off the stems, making it easy to remove the stems themselves prior to blending.

2 cups nondairy milk	2 cloves garlic, minced
2½ cups vegetable broth	4 sprigs thyme
1 small head cauliflower, roughly chopped	Himalayan pink salt
	Freshly ground black pepper
3–4 Yukon gold potatoes, peeled and chopped	½ cup cashews
	½ cup water
1 small onion, chopped	Chopped fresh chives for serving

- Combine the milk, broth, cauliflower, potatoes, onion, garlic, and thyme in a large soup pot.
- Season with salt and pepper.
- Bring to a boil and then simmer, covered, until the veggies are tender, about 18 to 20 minutes.
- In a high-speed blender, add the cashews and water and blend until perfectly smooth and creamy.
- Set aside.
- Once the veggies in the pot are done, remove and discard the thyme stems.
- Blend the soup in batches with the cashew cream until it is all perfectly creamy and well mixed in the soup pot.
- Adjust the flavor with salt and pepper.
- Garnish with a sprinkle of chives.

Pasta with Tofu, Broccolini, and Zucchini

This is one of our regular weekly meals. We switch off between tofu and chickpeas. Occasionally, we'll switch up the vegetable, too—e.g., do zucchini only, or broccolini only, or peas. Asparagus works great as well . . .

½ brick super-firm or nagari tofu, cubed	2 bunches broccolini, roughly chopped
1 tablespoon tamari	1 zucchini, cubed (optional)
1 tablespoon vegetable bouillon (preferably Better Than Bouillon Seasoned Vegetable Base)	1 pound whole-grain (e.g. quinoa, whole wheat, brown rice) spiral or penne pasta
½ onion, diced	¼ cup soy or hemp milk
¼ cup white wine or water	2 tablespoons nutritional yeast

- In a 11-by-13-inch nonstick pan, sauté the cubed tofu in tamari until browned, about 5 minutes.
- Add the bouillon and continue sautéing, about 5 to 10 minutes longer.
- Add the onion and sauté until translucent, about 5 minutes.
- Add the white wine and/or water.
- Add the broccolini and sauté until slightly soft, about 5 to 10 minutes.
- Add the zucchini (optional) and continue to sauté, adding more liquid as needed.
- Prepare the pasta per package instructions, drain, rinse, and return to the pot.
- Add the soy or hemp milk and nutritional yeast to the pasta and mix.
- Add the tofu-broccolini-zucchini mixture to the pasta, stirring thoroughly until well mixed.

BBQ Baked Tofu with Mashed Potatoes and Braised Greens

Talk about comfort food. This is one of our weekend recipes. Really easy to do, but does take a little more time than others. The BBQ tofu makes for excellent sandwiches the next day! You can also make this with portobello mushrooms–simply slice some portobellos, grill or pan-sear them, and cover with BBQ sauce!

BBQ TOFU

1 brick extra-firm tofu, pressed and sliced into ¼-inch-thick slices
⅛ cup lemon juice
⅛ cup tamari
¼ cup water
1–2 teaspoons extra-virgin olive oil (optional)
⅛ cup white wine (optional)
1 bottle BBQ sauce (preferably low-oil, low-sugar)

- Preheat the oven to 400°F.
- Layer the sliced tofu in a baking pan, spreading the pieces apart as much as possible.
- In a mixing bowl, combine the lemon juice, tamari, water, and olive oil and white wine, if using, and whisk together until well mixed.
- Pour the liquid mixture over the tofu, coating as much as possible.
- Place the baking pan in the oven and bake for 15 to 20 minutes. The tofu should reach a fairly firm texture and begin to brown.
- When the tofu is somewhat browned, remove the baking pan from the oven and pour the BBQ sauce on the tofu, spreading with a brush or fork until well coated—typically, about half the bottle.
- Return the tofu to the oven and continue baking until it is chewy and well cooked.

MASHED POTATOES

4 large russet potatoes (about 1 ½ pounds)
2 garlic cloves, peeled and smashed
Unsweetened nondairy milk (e.g., soy, almond, hemp)
1 teaspoon garlic powder
1 teaspoon onion powder
Salt and pepper to taste

- Peel the potatoes and cut into quarters.
- In a large pot, cover the potatoes with water.
- Bring the water to a boil, then reduce to a simmer.
- Simmer the potatoes until soft throughout. (Test by pushing a knife through the center of the potato.)
- Drain the potatoes, then mash.
- Add the nondairy milk and mix thoroughly.
- Add salt and pepper to taste.

BRAISED GREENS

2 bunches dinosaur kale, chard, collards, or a mixture of all three, roughly chopped
Approximately ½–1 cup vegetable broth

- Combine the chopped greens and a little vegetable broth together in a pot.
- Bring to medium heat and continue moving the greens around until softened to taste, about 5 to 10 minutes.
- Serve warm with the tofu and mashed potatoes.

ROASTED SEASONAL VEGETABLES SOUP

One of my favorite winter recipes. Another great option is simply to roast the vegetables and serve them over quinoa, brown rice, buckwheat, or wild rice. Very easy to grab whatever veggies you have in the fridge, cut them up, roast them, and go for it.

ROASTED SEASONAL VEGETABLES

1 cup beets (red or yellow), cut into chunks

1 cup carrots, cut into chunks

1 cup sweet potato, cut into chunks

1 cup potato, cut into chunks

1 cup of seasonal vegetable of your choice (i.e., celery, zucchini or squash), cut into chunks

Spray oil

1–3 teaspoons thyme and/or rosemary

½ teaspoon salt

¼ teaspoon black pepper

CASHEW CREAM

1 cup cashews

¼ cup nutritional yeast

2 cups water

1 tablespoon lemon juice or golden balsamic vinegar

1 teaspoon Ume plum vinegar

1 teaspoon miso paste

2–3 cups vegetable stock, as needed

Chives and/or parsley, minced

To prepare the vegetables:
- Place the cut vegetables on sheet pans in a single layer, taking care not to overcrowd.
- Spray lightly with oil, and mix until evenly coated.
- Sprinkle the herbs and salt and pepper over the vegetables and mix until evenly coated.
- Bake in the oven at 425°F for 10 minutes.
- Flip the vegetables over with a spatula and cook 10 more minutes or until golden brown and/or fork-tender.

To make the cashew cream:
- Combine all the cashew-cream ingredients in a blender and blend until smooth.
- Transfer the cashew cream to a separate bowl and set aside.

To make the soup:
- Using a high-speed blender, blend the prepared roasted vegetables in multiple small batches with enough vegetable stock to blend until smooth. Begin by just covering each batch of vegetables in the blender with the stock, then adding more stock as needed to reach creamy consistency as you blend.
- As each batch is blended, transfer to a soup pot until all roasted vegetables are blended.
- Place the soup pot on the stove and begin to heat, stirring occasionally.
- Add the cashew cream and salt, pepper, and additional thyme and/or rosemary to taste.
- Bring the soup to a simmer.
- Serve hot and garnish with chives and/or parsley.

LISA'S LENTIL SOUP

A pressure cooker rocks on this recipe (see the resources section), but a good ol' soup pot works just fine, too . . .

1–2 teaspoons olive oil or vegetable stock

2 onions, chopped

6 cloves garlic, minced

2 tablespoons fresh rosemary, chopped

1 bay leaf

Cayenne pepper to taste (optional)

½ cup rinsed quinoa

1 (14½-ounce) can whole tomatoes

10 cups vegetable stock made with Better Than Bouillon Seasoned
   Vegetable Base

2 cups French or green lentils

4 cups lightly packed fresh baby spinach

Salt and pepper to taste

Stovetop directions:

- Add the olive oil or vegetable stock to a preheated heavy stockpot.
- Add the onions, and sauté until translucent, about 3 to 5 minutes.
- Stir in the garlic, rosemary, bay leaf, and cayenne, if using, and sauté for 2 to 3 more minutes.
- Stir in the quinoa.
- Sauté over medium heat for 5 minutes, or until the quinoa is lightly toasted and the onions are golden brown.
- Stir the tomatoes into the quinoa with the juice from the can.
- Add the stock and lentils.
- Bring to a simmer over high heat.
- Decrease the heat to medium-low, cover, and simmer, stirring occasionally, for 25 minutes or until the lentils are tender.

- Stir in the spinach until just tender.
- Add salt and pepper.
- Simmer 2 minutes longer, or until the spinach wilts.
- Discard the bay leaf and season to taste with additional salt and pepper as needed.

Pressure-cooker directions:
- Sauté the onion, garlic, rosemary, and bay leaf in oil or vegetable stock until the onions are translucent.
- Add the rinsed lentils and quinoa.
- Sauté for approximately 1 minute.
- Add 6 teaspoons of Better Than Bouillon Seasoned Vegetable Base with 8 cups of water.
- Add the rest of the ingredients except the spinach.
- Lock the lid and set to 20 minutes of low pressure for French lentils or 14 minutes for green lentils, with 10 minutes of natural release.
- Release the remaining pressure and remove the lid.
- Add 2 more cups of water and about 3 teaspoons of bouillon and stir.
- Add salt and black pepper to taste. (*Note:* Beware of additional salt, as the bouillon is salty already.)
- Stir in the spinach and continue heating until it is wilted.

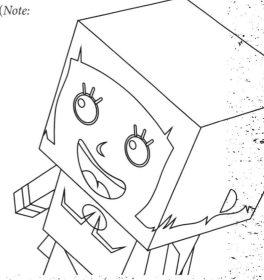

ALFREDO'S PASTA

Notice that there's no oil in this recipe, and then notice how frickin' good it is. Combine this with whole-grain pastas and a salad, and good night.

2 cups raw cashews

2 cups water

3 tablespoons white miso paste

1 teaspoon garlic powder

1 teaspoon freshly ground black pepper

¼ cup white cooking wine

1 tablespoon nutritional yeast

1 teaspoon salt (you may want to mix blender ingredients without salt and add
  to taste, since miso pastes can vary in saltiness)

1 pound whole-grain pasta

- Combine all ingredients except the white wine
  in a high-speed blender.
- Blend until fully smooth.
- Adjust the flavoring by adjusting the ingredients (miso, nutritional
  yeast), adding more salt and pepper as needed.
- Pour the mixture into a saucepan.
- Over medium heat, whisk the white wine into the mixture.
- Whisk continuously until the sauce starts to thicken and is heated
  through, about 5 to 7 minutes.
- If necessary, add more salt, pepper, and/or nutritional yeast to taste,
  mixing thoroughly.
- Prepare the pasta per package instructions and toss with the sauce.

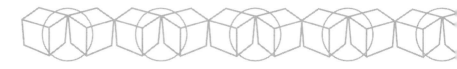

VEGGIE SANDWICHES OR WRAPS
(A CREATE-YOUR-OWN MEAL)

I love the simple, and a veggie sandwich or wrap is just that. My kids devour these (well, more specifically, devour mine, then ask for their own). Great for quick lunches, or snacks.

Nori sheets (raw preferred, but toasted fine)
Lisa's Cashew Ranch Dressing (page 171) or Tahini Dressing (page 176)
Tomato, thinly sliced in half-moons
Cucumber, sliced lengthwise, then cut into thin strips
Avocado, thinly sliced
Red onion, thinly sliced in half-moons
Carrot, shredded (optional)
Bell pepper, thinly sliced into strips (optional)
Hot sauce and/or salsa (optional)

- Lay out the nori sheets on a cutting board or counter.
- Spread approximately 1 tablespoon of the cashew ranch dressing down each sheet on the diagonal.
- Lay approximately equal amounts of the different veggies, depending on personal preference.
- Add hot sauce or salsa to taste.
- Fold in corners over approximately 1 inch of the dressing/veggies.
- Roll the sheet, tucking ingredients in as you go, to create a tight, sealed roll.

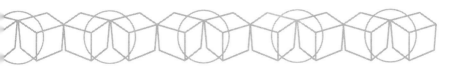

"Don't Be Afraid of Potatoes" Potatoes
(A CREATE-YOUR-OWN MEAL)

Check out my "Fear the Potato" video on my YouTube channel, but I (and most people I know) love potatoes. They're great, filling, and an easy medium to top with delicious toppings to create your own custom meal. Throw a salad on the side, and it's a meal. Yes, potatoes and salad are a frickin' meal.

Oh, potatoes, why do so many people argue about you?

I LOVE potatoes. Sweet, Russet, Yukon. Bring 'em on. Heavy-box, delicious, and satisfying.

Why the bad rap?

An unfounded fear of "carbs." This is a healthy carbohydrate, and, frankly, what ruins potatoes nutritionally is what people put on them. Butter, sour cream, and Bac-Os on the potato? Right, the carbs are the problem. Come on!

Instead, frickin' enjoy potatoes . . . Bake, roast, mash away. Toppings? Salsa, baked beans, chili beans, or, this incredible cashew ranch dressing (see recipe that follows—it makes a phenomenal salad dressing and dip, too).

Serve with a big salad, and you've got some serious nutrition under your belt. Literally.

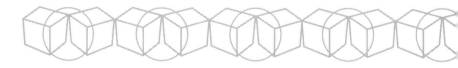

LISA'S CASHEW RANCH DRESSING

2 cups cashews

2¼ cup filtered water

3 tablespoons lemon juice (approximately ½ lemon)

2 tablespoons apple-cider vinegar

1 teaspoon garlic powder

3 teaspoons onion powder

2 teaspoons dill

1 teaspoon dried basil

½ teaspoon freshly ground black pepper or more to taste

Salt to taste

- Blend all ingredients until creamy and smooth. If too thick, add more water.
- Store in the refrigerator. (*Note:* The dressing will thicken in the refrigerator. Simply add a little more water as needed to thin before subsequent uses.)

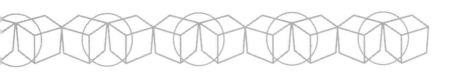

Easy Veggie Stir-Fry

This is one of those "what the heck are we going to have for dinner?" dinners. Easy and quick—use what you have, and enjoy.

2 tablespoons agave nectar

¼ cup soy sauce

⅛ cup water

1–2 teaspoon cornstarch (optional)

1–2 teaspoons olive or coconut oil
  or vegetable stock

10–15 cremini mushrooms, sliced

1 green bell pepper, chopped

1 red bell pepper, chopped

1 cup broccoli florets

2 carrots, chopped

1 cup green beans, ends removed

Bamboo shoots (optional)

2 cups cooked brown rice or quinoa

- Mix the agave, soy sauce, water, and cornstarch, if using. Set aside.
- Heat a frying pan or wok over medium-high heat, then add the oil or vegetable stock.
- If using oil, move the pan around until it is well coated by the oil, then pour off the excess oil.
- Add the mushrooms, bell peppers, broccoli, carrots, green beans, and bamboo shoots, if using.
- Mix around using a spatula until warmed.
- Put a lid on the frying pan/wok and let the vegetables cook for 4 to 5 minutes.
- Toss the vegetables and continue cooking uncovered for another 2 minutes.
- Add the agave-soy-water mixture.
- Continue stirring until the vegetables are cooked but still a bit firm (al dente), about 5 minutes.
- Serve over brown rice and/or quinoa.

Veggie Burger Tostadas

My wife, Lisa, invented these. We use Sunshine burgers, and we know that not all veggie burgers are created alike. Sunshine's ingredients are heavy-box, and taste great . . .

Sunshine Burgers, Dr. Praeger's Veggie Burgers, or homemade veggie burger
Small corn tortillas
Daiya cheese (or any nondairy cheese)
Ketchup
Mustard

- In a large nonstick pan, heat the veggie burgers until hot, flipping intermittently.
- Lay the corn tortillas on a cutting board or counter.
- Cut the heated veggie burgers into approximately ½-inch-wide strips.
- Squirt a small strip of ketchup and mustard down the middle of each corn tortilla.
- Place the veggie burger strips on top of the ketchup/mustard.
- Top each tortilla/veggie burger with shredded nondairy cheese.
- Place the completed tortillas on a parchment paper–lined baking sheet or baking pan.
- Place under the broiler, and broil on low until the cheese is melted and the tortillas are hot, about 5 to 10 minutes.

Real Burritos

Who doesn't love a big, honkin' burrito? 'Nuff said.

1 bunch kale, chopped

½ onion, chopped

Vegetable broth, stock, or bouillon

4 whole-grain burrito wraps or tortillas, warmed

2 cups cooked brown rice or quinoa

1 (15-ounce can) of black or pinto beans, drained and rinsed

TOPPINGS

Salsa

Lettuce, shredded

Nondairy cheese

Tomatoes, chopped

Green onions, sliced

Pickled onions

Cilantro, chopped

Avocado, sliced

Hot sauce

Fresh jalapeno or serrano peppers, chopped

- In a saucepan, sauté the kale and onions in the veggie broth until soft, about 5 to 7 minutes.
- In a warm tortilla, place the kale/onion sauté, brown rice or quinoa, and beans and any or all of the toppings!

PIZZA NIGHT
(*A CREATE-YOUR-OWN MEAL*)

As with Falafel Night, my family loves Pizza Night. We buy premade, whole-grain pizza rounds, and the kids make their own (with heavy-box toppings, of course). Is it better to make your own dough? Yes. But, seriously, what am I, a fancy lad?

Whole-grain flatbreads or pizza rounds
Marinara sauce and/or pesto (recipe follows)
Assorted toppings—sliced tomato, olives, minced garlic, sliced onion, jalapeño, sliced mushrooms, nondairy cheese, etc.

- Top flatbreads or pizza rounds with desired sauces and ingredients.
- Bake at 450°F until well cooked (or, alternatively, follow baking directions on the flatbread/pizza-round packages), about 8 to 10 minutes.

PESTO

2 cups fresh basil leaves, chopped, or 1 cup chopped basil and
  1 cup chopped kale
¾ cup walnuts
¼–½ cup nutritional yeast
2 tablespoons olive oil or water
6–8 cloves garlic, roughly chopped
1 tablespoon white or brown rice miso
1 teaspoon black pepper
Salt to taste

- Place all ingredients into a food processor and process until smooth, adding more water as needed to reach desired consistency.

FALAFEL NIGHT!
(A CREATE-YOUR-OWN MEAL)

One of our favorite weekend meals, and our kids love them. We lay out the heavy-box toppings, and they build their own . . .

1 box Fantastic World Foods Falafel Mix

8 tortillas (whole wheat, whole grain gluten-free, and/or corn)

Hummus (we love Sabra brand, but look for a hummus with simple ingredients)

2 tomatoes, chopped

1 avocado, sliced

5 leaves of lettuce, shredded

½ cup Kalamata olives, chopped

¼ jar sliced pepperoncini

½–1 cup Tahini Dressing

TAHINI DRESSING

1 cup raw or toasted sesame tahini

½ teaspoon marjoram

½ teaspoon paprika

½ teaspoon oregano

1 tablespoon ume plum vinegar or ½ teaspoon salt to taste

1–2 tablespoon lemon juice

Filtered water until desired consistency and flavor

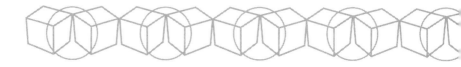

To prepare the falafel patties:

- Make the falafel patties according to the instructions on the package, using the broil option as directed (in lieu of frying in oil).

To make the tahini dressing:

- In a mixing bowl, combine all the ingredients and whisk or fork the mix together until well combined. The mixture will initially become granular in consistency; continue whisking until smooth.
- Depending on desired consistency (e.g., thinner for salad dressing, thicker for dip or falafel sauce), add more water and/or lemon juice as needed, continuing to whisk.

To assemble the falafels:

- Lay a tortilla flat on a plate.
- Spread a layer of hummus across the middle of the tortilla from end to end.
- Break up the falafel patty along the hummus.
- Place pieces of tomato, avocado, lettuce, Kalamata olives, and pepperoncini in layers on top of the falafel
- Drizzle tahini dressing over all other ingredients.
- Roll the tortilla like a burrito.

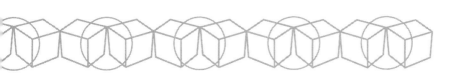

LENTIL "MEAT" BALLS

These are easy to prepare and can be enjoyed in a variety of ways: over spaghetti with store-bought or homemade sauce, on dairy-free sandwich bread as a meatless meatball sub, in a wrap, or on their own.

2 cups red lentils, rinsed

3 cups vegetable stock

½ cup finely chopped onions

3 cloves garlic, finely chopped

8 ounces or approximately 3 cups cremini mushrooms, sliced

1 tablespoon dried thyme

1 tablespoon dried oregano

1 tablespoon ground fennel seed

Approximately ¼ cup white wine

1–2 teaspoons vegetable bouillon

1 cup finely ground flax seeds

1 cup nutritional yeast

Approximately ¼ cup gluten-free flour (e.g., sorghum or rice flour) or whole-wheat pastry flour

Salt and freshly ground pepper to taste

- In a medium-large pot, combine the lentils, vegetable stock, onions, and garlic.
- Bring to a boil.
- Reduce heat and simmer covered for about 20 to 25 minutes or until very soft.
- Remove from heat and mash well with a potato masher or a fork.
- Set aside.
- Sauté mushrooms, thyme, oregano, and fennel in white wine and bouillon until mushrooms are soft, about 10 to 15 minutes.
- In a food processor or blender, combine half of the lentil mixture with the mushrooms, ground flax seeds, and nutritional yeast, then blend until smooth.
- Add the processed mixture to the remaining lentil mixture and mix with a wooden spoon until well mixed.
- Gradually stir in the sorghum or rice flour, 1 tablespoon at a time, until the mixture holds together.

- Adjust seasoning and add salt and pepper to taste.
- Allow the mixture to reach room temperature before forming into balls.
- Place the balls on a baking sheet and bake at 425°F for 30 to 40 minutes or until browned.

TACO NIGHT
(*A CREATE-YOUR-OWN MEAL*)

This is a great regular weekly meal. Plus, Lisa and I will make extra refried beans and quinoa to use in our next day's Big Frickin' Salads.

2 cups cooked quinoa or brown rice
1 can refried or whole beans
Tomatoes, chopped
Lettuce, shredded
Avocados, chopped
Red or yellow onion, chopped
Nondairy cheese shreds
Whole grain, tortillas, or wraps (whole-wheat tortillas, whole-grain gluten-free wraps, corn tortillas), warmed
Salsa

- Place portions of each ingredients on a plate for each person, with warmed tortillas on the side.
- Each person builds their own soft tacos to taste!

FREQUENTLY ASKED QUESTIONS

What follows are some questions I've received after giving talks on raising healthy and happy children.

- "We're trying to eat healthier. What do we do when our children go to birthday parties?"
    - There are a couple ways to handle this. 1) Remember, your MOTT is the name of the game, meaning that a party isn't going to break the bank. It's a few hours, tops. If your family eats well most of the time, don't sweat the special occasions. 2) The other option is to send healthier treats with your children. Because my family is plant based, we will often send them with their own treats that they get to pick out. These days, however, more parents are providing plant-based options at their children's parties—but we never, ever ask or expect. Side note: The treats we send are usually pretty light-box. (Plant based doesn't automatically mean healthy. Jolly Ranchers are jolly, to be sure . . . just not healthy.) Again, don't sweat the one-offs. In a world of increasing dairy and nut allergies, it's not exactly crazy to send your child with a bit of food.
- "What about healthy lunches at school?"
    - Making your child's lunch means you're in charge of how heavy-box they are. As with the regular weekly-menu concept above, I suggest a semiregular lunch. We keep the lunch choices minimal so we don't spend a ton of time making lunches each morning. Suggestions: box soups (many have quality ingredients); sandwiches on whole-

grain bread with almond butter, avocado, sliced tomato, and lettuce, etc.; whole grain crackers; cut veggies with cashew ranch dressing (see page 171); fruit.

Note: I have taught and worked with many parents who avoid feeding their children fruit for fear of sugar. Remember, it's what comes with the sugar (sugar=carbohydrate) that counts. Fruit has a ton of micronutrients, water and fiber. It's awesome. Let your children eat fruit!

- "I'm concerned because my child eats differently than other kids. I don't want him/her to feel self-conscious. What do I do?"
  - As a culture, we tend to place so much importance on food, making it a way bigger deal than it should be. It's just food, for crying out loud. Nevertheless, children will notice what another child eats, especially if it's starkly different. Fact is, however, most children don't come to school with the exact same lunch, and furthermore, no two children are alike. Understand (and explain to your child) that a ton of factors and behaviors define us. Your child is already different from other kids no matter what you feed them. Champion this, and keep the conversation alive about why you are eating the way you do. Since when is being different a bad thing?

- "My spouse is totally uninterested in teaching the kids healthy habits, and sometimes even tries to undo what I am teaching them. What do I do?"
  - This comes up all the time at my talks. A parent tells me she is struggling to feed the family well because her spouse/partner is not only *not* on board with the foods she is introducing, but in some cases is even going out of the way to derail the process by sneaking in the very foods she is trying to minimize. And so . . . here are my thoughts on

this. First of all, I am not a marriage counselor (remember Randy the Mechanic?). With that said, your family's health and happiness is of supreme importance and needs to be the highest priority for both parents. Communication between you and your spouse is key. But so is doing whatever it takes for the good of your children, so be open to marriage counseling. Having both parents on the same page works best for a family in every regard.

- "How do I handle negative comments from extended family and people in general?"
  - It blows my mind how many people feel the need to throw in their two cents without being asked. It's a tough spot when family members, friends, or even people we barely know criticize how we eat and/or live. As if our personal choices are somehow a judgment or critique of someone else. Unfortunately, that someone else can go on the attack because they feel judged. One solution? Do not engage. Change the subject. You won't change their minds anyway and shouldn't have to defend yourself. Instead, focus on the steps you are undertaking. Keep improving. Just as the example you set influences your children above all else, so, too, will it influence others. However, if pressed and/or you feel the need to defend yourself (why, oh why don't you eat bacon?!?), be honest and forthright—you are choosing to take better care of yourself and your family because it makes you happier. That is a fact. How they interpret *your* decisions has absolutely nothing to do with you. As my childhood friend would say, "It ain't in your movie."

- "What should I do if my child is overweight?"
  - I think any discussion of weight is irrelevant and damaging. Stay clear of any discussion about your child's

weight. The heavier-box your children eat over time, the healthier their bodies will be. As the body gets healthier, the weight gets healthier. That's how it works. What every child needs is love, care, protection, and nourishment. Add in more heavy-box food, improve your MOTT, and their bodies and minds will respond in kind.

- "I've heard from so many people that eating healthy is expensive! What if we have a limited budget?"
  - The fact that a crappy TV dinner often costs less than a couple of heads of organic lettuce is because our current food/political system (with subsidies, etc.) is insane. As a result, prices of subsidized foods are way cheaper than what those foods would cost without the subsidies. In other words, if it were a fair playing field, light-box food prices would soar. Since I don't see this changing any time soon (until I'm elected president, that is), here are my thoughts on the cost of healthy eating:

    1. When you (correctly) assess the health of a food not by the calories (i.e., protein/fat/carbohydrates) but by the micronutrients (vitamins, minerals, etc.), the argument that eating healthy is more expensive loses steam. Why? Because the fact that a cucumber is more expensive than an order of large fries makes sense—you are getting way more for your money with the cucumber. It's like complaining that a Ferrari is more expensive than a Chevy Nova. Of course, it's more expensive. It's a better car. Eating healthy costs more because you get more.
    2. When you factor in the side effects of eating a mostly light-box diet, eating heavier-box comes out on top. In other words, a diet of light-box foods typically

means more money spent on prescription and over-the-counter drugs (e.g., Tylenol, Pepto-Bismol, etc.) and even skin-care/hair-care products. The heavier-box your diet, the less money you end up spending on products you'd otherwise need to minimize/mitigate symptoms that come from a poor diet (headaches, inflammatory pain, low energy/fatigue, pimples, rashes, dry hair/skin, etc.).

3. It is possible to stay mostly heavy-box and reduce your grocery costs significantly. Brown rice, quinoa, buckwheat, oats, and dried beans are all affordable. If you can't afford organic, buy conventional. Conventional fruits and vegetables, whole grains, beans, nuts, and seeds are still healthy. If possible, steer clear of the "dirty dozen" (conventionally grown apples, bell peppers, celery, cherries, grapes, nectarines, peaches, pears, potatoes, strawberries, spinach, and tomatoes [source: the Environmental Working Group: ewg. org]), as well as conventionally grown corn, soy, and wheat. Raw nuts tend to be expensive, but I recommend a relatively small daily amount anyway, so no need to buy substantial amounts of these.

4. Preparing your own meals keeps costs down. And if you follow my suggestion by creating a regular recurring meal plan, you save money *and* time.

- "I'm so frickin' motivated to get my family going on this, and I want to go BIG! Should I blow off Small Stepping and just have at it?"
  - ° Hold on there a minute, Sparky. First, if you burn yourself and your family out by taking on too much, you'll lose everything you've worked for. Take a bit of time before

you pull the trigger to settle on a low-stress starting point. Remember, you are in charge of your Steps List, so if you really are motivated and don't perceive the transition to be stressful, go ahead and ramp up! But don't forget that not everyone's Small Steps are necessarily the same size. A step is small if you can do it without upset. So, if you can handle going BIG, then, by golly, BIG is your Small Step.

- "Sid, so I guess you think you're the perfect parent, since you wrote this book?"
  - Not by a long shot. But my wife and I understand this: No matter how hard we try to be excellent parents, no matter how correct we think our parenting is, we will make mistakes. At the same time, we hope that we empower our children to take good care of themselves and eventually, if they become parents, improve on the areas where we fell short. I want any parent reading this to understand the "practice" that is parenting. It is an ongoing learning process that, frankly, lasts as long as you do. Love your children. Show them you're doing your best. Know that by making yourself stronger, you are making them stronger.

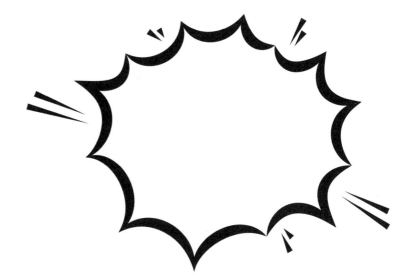

GLOSSARY

For those of you who might jump around this book in a, let's say, nonlinear fashion, there are a few terms you might come across that could confuse you. Here is a mini-glossary to help.

MOTT: Most Of The Time. I believe your health and happiness are determined by what you do most of the time, not necessarily all of the time. Looking at health/happiness this way is crucial when it comes to subjects like food, where people can, upon learning what constitutes a healthy diet, become militant and rigid. When it comes to children, the fact is that a little bit of less-than-healthy food once in a while isn't going to break the bank. Focus on improving what you and your family do and eat most of the time, and you won't sweat the one-offs.

Heavy-Box and Light-Box Foods: I write about physical nutrition (e.g., how we move and feed our bodies) and mental nutrition (e.g., how we feed our minds—entertainment, socializing, creativity) in terms of gift boxes: light boxes and heavy boxes. Every gift has wrapping paper, but the value of a gift is determined by what is inside. Food is the same way. A Twinkie and a cucumber both provide our bodies with energy (that is, the wrapping paper: protein, fat, carbohydrate), but the cucumber is a heavier box because of what comes with the energy it provides (that is, what is inside the box: vitamins, minerals, phytochemicals, antioxidants, fibers, water). The heavier the box, the more substance; the lighter, the less. Same goes for mental nutrition. Both reality TV shows and *War and Peace* entertain us, but one is clearly a lighter box than the other. In this book, and in my practice, I don't advocate completely giving up light-box nutrition—rather, I recommend creating a balance of heavy and light boxes that works for you.

Me/Not Me Game: This is a game I invented that works incredibly well for parents and nonparents alike. My Small Steps system involves first and foremost getting to know who you truly are regardless of how you may have been behaving. In other words, I argue that someone who is not healthy but wants to be healthy is actually a healthy person who just hasn't been acting in line with who they are. The game involves taking a few moments here and there to identify which of your actions represent the real you— and which do not. By playing it, you find out who you are and what you stand for. The game removes shame, guilt, and negative self-criticism and replaces them with more knowledge and a clear direction of how you want your life to be. How to get there? My Small Steps approach. What the heck are Small Steps, you ask? Good question…

Small Steps: My version of a Small Step is any new behavior someone can incorporate into their lives with minimal stress. For example, if someone wants to start exercising for the first time in their lives, his/her Small Step might be a one minute walk around the house. Whatever gets the ball rolling and enables one to easily pull off the new behavior Most Of The Time. (See what I did there? Brought the MOTT into the conversation. Full circle. Boom.) The most common misconception of my approach, however, is that the size of an anyone's Small Step is the same for everyone. Not so. For example, someone who has exercised a ton in the past and wants to start up again may have the small step of a one-mile jog around the neighborhood, while, for the person mentioned above, the small step may be a one-minute walk around the house. The size of the small step is whatever gets someone going on a new behavior with minimal stress, no dread, and (ideally) fun.

Wall of Behaviors: I refer to our existing habits and routines as our "wall of behaviors." I argue that if you try and cram a new behavior in the wall by taking on too much too soon, you will most likely fail. The wall will kick it back out. On the other hand, if you ease your way in, making little cracks in the wall (with eating healthier, exercising, painting, meditating, writing, or anything new) *and* stick with it long enough, your wall will incorporate the new habit or routine.

RESOURCES

Full disclosure: I am financially connected to two of the resources that follow, and I placed them first so there is no confusion. All other recommendations—books, apps, products—are those I stand behind but in which I have absolutely no financial stake whatsoever . . .

I hope you give my regular-weekly-meals model a try, but the cookbooks I recommend are great, fun, and perfect for hunting down new or replacement recipes to fit into that regular schedule.

Sid (intentionally referring to myself in third person) is financially connected to:

- Health Made Simple
  - Matt Frazier (who wrote the foreword to this book), the No Meat Athlete, and I created this meal plan to teach people how easy it is to eat a healthy diet. The site consists of multiple 30-day meal plans with recipes, instructional videos, nutritional guidance, live Q&As, and more. It's super affordable, and Matt and I are very proud of what we created . . .
- SmallSteppers.com
  - This is my own site that I created to teach people the ins and outs of my Small Steps System. It is a twelve-week program, start to finish. You get in, learn the system, and get out. Weekly videos, daily e-mails, live Q&As, and more.

Sid (still hangin' in third person) is *not* financially connected to:

- Pressure Cookers
  - I know it's shocking, but I'm not financially connected to pressure cookers. However . . . we've been using a pressure cooker for years now and love it. I highly recommend buying an electric version (i.e., not a stove-top model). Ours,

a Cuisinart, is still going strong after eight years. Great for soups, the lentil meatballs, quinoa, beans, brown rice, and a ton more. Load it up, turn it on, and walk away (toward your nearest family member to hang out).

- Aida
  - ∘ This is the app I use for my integrated exercise reminders. It's fairly customizable. I have mine set to go off on the hour between 11 AM and 5 PM, Monday through Friday. I've set the alarm to say, "Push-ups and/or squats," but that's just me.
- Wunderlist
  - ∘ This is an awesome app to use for your Steps List.
- *Lynda's Healing Kitchen: Life Lessons, Love, and Recipes,* by Lynda Layng
  - ∘ Lynda is a private chef and a super-great person, and it shows in her recipes.
- *The No Meat Athlete Cookbook: Whole Food, Plant-Based Recipes to Fuel Your Workouts—and the Rest of Your Life,* by Matt Frazier and Stepfanie Romine
  - ∘ This is Matt's cookbook, and he did not ask me to include it here. It's a great book for athletes and nonathletes alike. Easy and healthy recipes.
- *This Cheese Is Nuts: Delicious Vegan Cheese at Home,* by Julie Piatt
  - ∘ Julie is a bud and a great chef, and I'm recommending this book purely for fun.
- *Forks Over Knives—The Cookbook: Over 300 Recipes for Plant-Based Eating All Through the Year,* by Del Sroufe
  - ∘ I had Del on my podcast—great story and great guy. These are heavy-box recipes, to be sure . . .

REFERENCES

Barnard, Neal D. *The Cheese Trap: How Breaking a Surprising Addiction Will Help You Lose Weight, Gain Energy, and Get Healthy* (New York: Hachette, 2017).

Chutkan, Robynne. *The Microbiome Solution: A Radical New Way to Heal Your Body from the Inside Out* (New York: Penguin, 2015).

Cottrell, Elizabeth C., Susan E. Ozanne. "Early Life Programming of Obesity and Metabolic Disease," *Physiology & Behavior*, Apr. 22, 2008, 94(1): 1728.

Davis, Garth. *Proteinaholic: How Our Obsession with Meat Is Killing Us and What We Can Do About It* (New York: HarperOne, 2015).

De Mello, Vanessa D., Jussi Paananen, Jaana Lindström, Maria A. Lankinen, Lin Shi, Johanna Kuusisto, Jussi Pihlajamäki, Seppo Auriola, Marko Lehtonen, Olov Rolandsson, Ingvar A. Bergdahl, Elise Nordin, Pirjo Ilanne-Parikka, Sirkka Keinänen-Kiukaanniemi, Rikard Landberg, Johan G. Eriksson, Jaakko Tuomilehto, Kati Hanhineva, Matti Uusitupa. "Indolepropionic Acid and Novel Lipid Metabolites Are Associated with a Lower Risk of Type 2 Diabetes in the Finnish Diabetes Prevention Study," *Scientific Reports*, 2017; 7: 46337.

Duhigg, Charles. *The Power of Habit: Why We Do What We Do in Life and Business* (New York: Random House, 2012).

Dweck, Carol S. *Mindset: The New Psychology of Success* (New York: Random House, 2006).

Fuhrman, Joel. *Disease Proof Your Child: Feeding Kids Right* (New York: St. Martin's Griffin, 2006).

Fuhrman, Joel. *Eat to Live: The Revolutionary Formula for Fast and Sustained Weight Loss* (Boston: Little, Brown, 2003).

Greger, Michael, and Gene Stone. *How Not to Die: Discover the Foods Scientifically Proven to Prevent and Reverse Disease* (New York: Flatiron, 2015).

Luby, Joan L., Deanna M. Barch, Andy Belden, Michael S. Gaffrey, Rebecca Tillman, Casey Babb, Tomoyuki Nishino, Hideo Suzuki, Kelly N. Botteron. "Maternal Support in Early Childhood Predicts Larger Hippocampal Volumes at School Age," *Proceedings of the National Academy of Sciences*, Feb. 21, 2012, 109(8): 2854–9.

O'Neil, Adrienne, Shae E. Quirk, Siobhan Housden, Sharon L. Brennan, Lana J. Williams, Julie A. Pasco, Michael Berk, and Felice N. Jacka. "Relationship Between Diet and Mental Health in Children and Adolescents: A Systematic Review," *American Journal of Public Health*, Oct. 2014, 104(10): 31–42.

Pina-Camacho, Laura, Sarah K. Jensen, Darya Gaysina, Edward D. Barker. "Maternal Depression Symptoms, Unhealthy Diet, and Child Emotional-Behavioural Dysregulation," *Psychological Medicine*, July 2015, 45(9): 1851–60.

Rao, Hengyi, Laura Betancourt, Joan M. Giannetta, Nancy L. Brodsky, Marc Korczykowski, Brian B. Avants, James C. Gee, Jiongjiong Wanga, Hallam Hurt, John A. Detre, Martha J. Farah. "Early Parental Care Is Important for Hippocampal Maturation: Evidence from Brain Morphology in Humans," *Neuroimage*, Jan 1, 2010, 49(1): 1144–50.

Sanchez, Marina, Shirin Panahi, and Angelo Tremblay. "Childhood Obesity: A Role for Gut Microbiota?" *International Journal of Environmental Research and Public Health*, Jan. 2015, 12(1): 162–175.

Selhub, Eva. "Nutritional Psychiatry: Your Brain on Food," Harvard Health Publications, Harvard Medical School, Nov. 16, 2015: http://www.health.harvard.edu/blog/nutritional-psychiatry-your-brain-on-food-201511168626.

Sonnenburg, Justin, and Erica Sonnenburg. *The Good Gut: Taking Control of Your Weight, Your Mood, and Your Long-Term Health.* (New York: Penguin, 2015).

Tuttle, Will. *World Peace Diet: Eating for Spiritual Health and Social Harmony* (Devon, UK: Lantern, 2004).

ACKNOWLEDGMENTS

Big ol' thanks to: Chris Gruener and everyone at Cameron + Company/ Roundtree for giving me another go 'round. • Jan Hughes, Cameron's managing editor, for not only being open to my 180-degree shift in this book's direction, but for laying down some great ideas and feedback. • Joan and Jeff Stanford, for their continued support, passion, compassion, unlimited espressos, and the resort lobby that proved to be incredibly conducive to writing. • Matt Frazier for writing the foreword and for his own good works. • My mom and dad, for providing a loving upbringing and home, and for their continued support and love. • My children, Luna, Rinah, and Rónán, for never-ending inspiration, fun, joy, and love. • Lisa, the love of my life, for everything.

Text copyright © 2018 Sid Garza-Hillman
Foreword copyright © 2018 Matt Frazier

Cover design by Iain R. Morris

Creative Director: Iain R. Morris   Designer: Rob Dolgaard

Editor: Jan Hughes   Copy editor: Mark Nichol

Proofreaders: Lucy Walker, Mason Harper

Library of Congress Cataloging-in-Publication Data available.
ISBN: 978-1-944903-21-3

10 9 8 7 6 5 4 3 2 1

Manufactured in the United States

Roundtree Press
149 Kentucky Street, Suite 7
Petaluma, CA 94952
www.roundtreepress.com